THE FAT BURN REVOLUTION

Note

While every effort has been made to ensure that the content of this book
is as technically accurate and as sound as possible, neither the author nor
the publishers can accept responsibility for any injury or loss sustained as
a result of the use of this material. All readers should seek medical
consult their doctor before commencing any exercise programme.

Published by Bloomsbury Publishing Plc

50 Bedford Square
London WC1B 3DP

www.bloomsbury.com

First edition 2014

Copyright © 2014 Julia Buckley

ISBN (print): 978-1-4081-9156-9
ISBN (edpf): 978-1-4081-9158-3
ISBN (epub): 978-1-4081-9157-6

Acknowledgements
Cover photograph © Grant Pritchard
Inside photographs © Grant Pritchard with the exception of the following;
pp. 36, 40, 43, 45, 49 © Shutterstock

Commissioning Editor: Kirsty Schaper
Editor: Sarah Cole
Design: Nimbus Design

This book is produced using paper that is made from wood grown in managed,
sustainable forests. It is natural, renewable and recyclable. The logging and
manufacturing processes conform to the environmental regulations of the
country of origin.

Typeset in 8pt on 11pt Bliss by Nimbus Design

Printed and bound in China by C&C Offset Printing Co

10 9 8 7 6 5 4 3 2 1

THE FAT BURN REVOLUTION

Julia Buckley

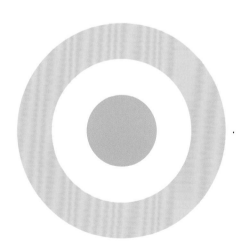

BLOOMSBURY

LONDON · NEW DELHI · NEW YORK · SYDNEY

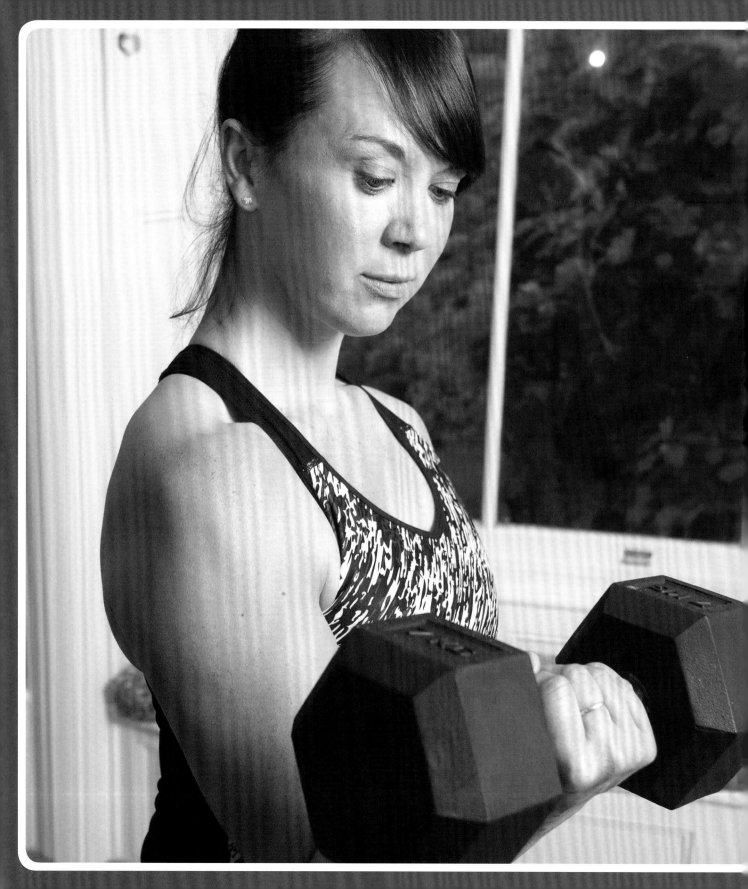

contents

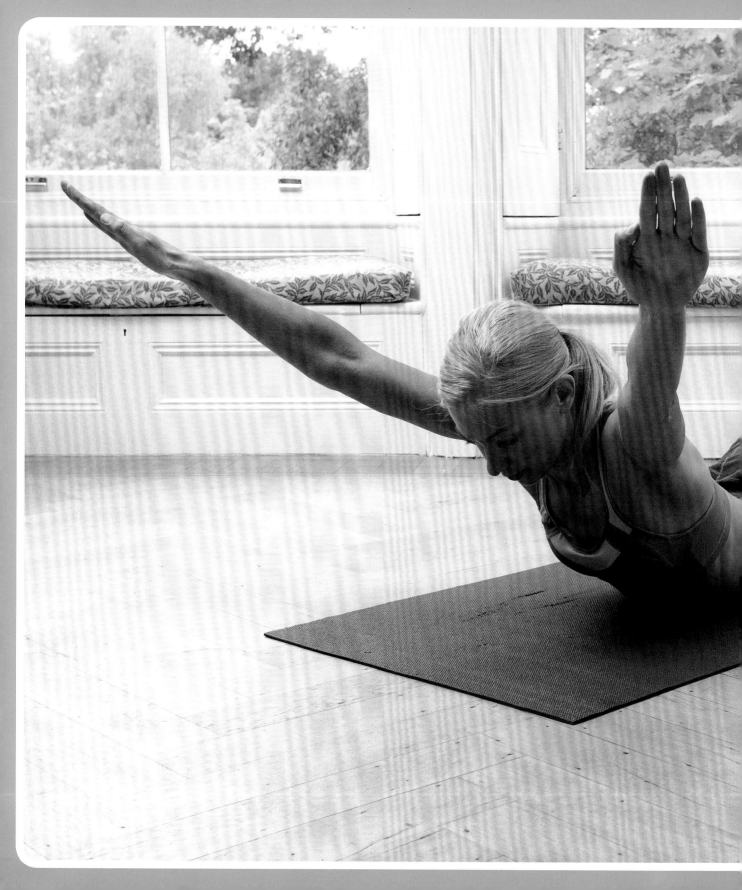

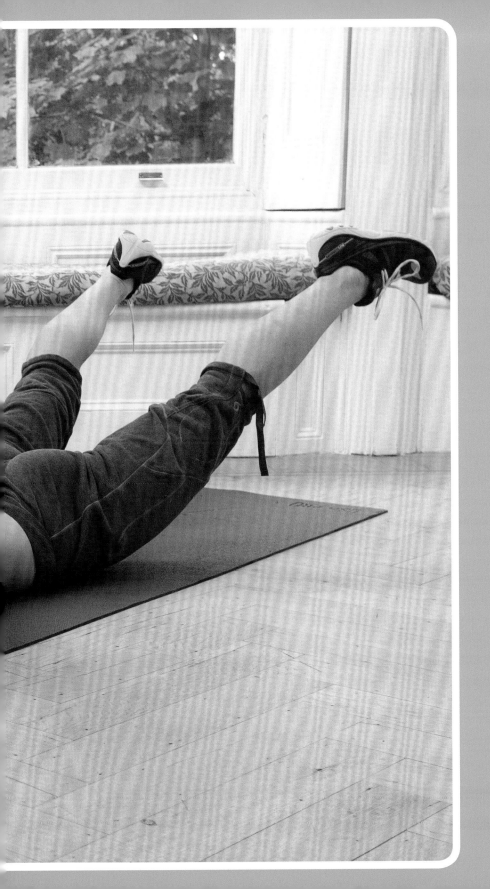

the **revolution** starts in the mind

the road to the
revolution

Welcome to the Fat Burn Revolution. My name is Julia and I am a fitness journalist and personal trainer. I devised this 12-week programme to enable you to get into outstanding physical condition and finally shed the excess fat that has dragged you down for way too long.

> If you have yet to experience being physically fit, get excited, you are in for something wonderful.

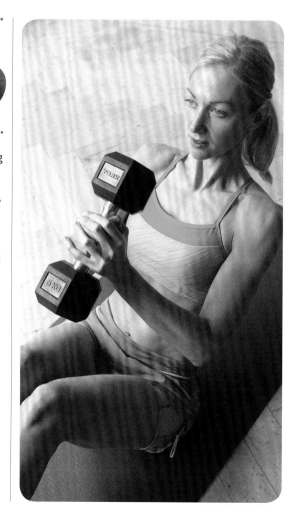

If you love exercise and thrive on the amazing feeling of being in great shape, you and I definitely have at least one thing in common. But if, on the other hand, you are not a typical fitness fanatic we have that in common too. I grew up hating playing sports. At school Physical Education was a horrible, humiliating experience where friends seemed to morph into vicious opponents or seething 'teammates'. The teachers in charge were no help. Their attitude was that you were either a talented sportsperson or you weren't. And if you weren't, they made no secret of the fact that you were a waste of their time. Unfortunately, I was well into the latter category.

It got almost to the point of a phobia. I've never admitted this publicly before, but in my last year at I school I used to pretend that the silver christening bangle I wore on my wrist was too small to fit over my hand and I couldn't take it off. Jewellery was

**It's never to late to start
exercising or to change the way
you train and improve your diet.**

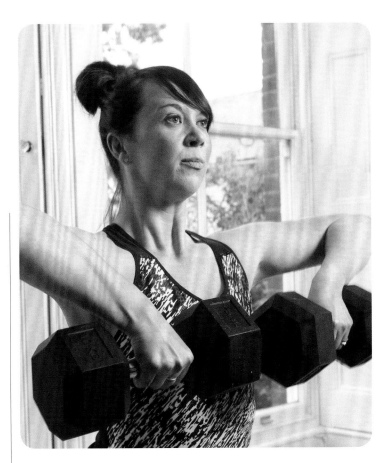

banned in PE class, so the teachers said I couldn't
join in unless I had it cut off. I refused, saying it was
sentimental. So instead of taking part in games, they
sat me at a desk in a corridor and made me copy out
the rulebook of a different sport each week. It was
supposed to be a punishment, but I was more than
happy with the arrangement – that indignity didn't
come close to the mortification of being the last girl
on the bench when teams were picked.

It was only a few days after I left school at 16
that I noticed my hand had grown and now the
bracelet would not come off. The irony. Without a
second thought, I took a pair of pliers from my dad's
toolbox and snapped through it. It almost felt like
cutting the chains that had tied to me to that lonely
shameful desk in the corridor – at last I didn't have
to do (or rather not do) PE any more.

I'm a very honest person by nature, and I'm
not proud to have lied back then. But I wanted to
admit my deception here to let you know that I do
understand what it's like to feel like a carthorse in
a dressage show. I want you to have no doubt that
not being a sports hero when you were growing up
does not mean you can't be fit as an adult. I am in
my mid-thirties now and in the best shape of my
life. And I'm happy to report that it is a phenomenal
feeling.

I also know what it is like to carry extra fat
around. I've never been more than a couple of
stone overweight, but my weight has fluctuated

> You have to push outside of your
> comfort zone if you want to change
> your body. Regular intense challenging
> workouts, supported by good nutrition,
> cause the body to respond and adapt.
> That's when changes happen.

throughout my life. Before I discovered the principles
and methods I'll share with you in this book, I
was locked in a constant battle to either get to or
maintain a body shape I felt happy with. I've also
worked with many people who have lost a lot more
weight. The Fat Burn Revolution programme has
made incredible and lasting changes to their lives.

I was in my late teens when I began to understand

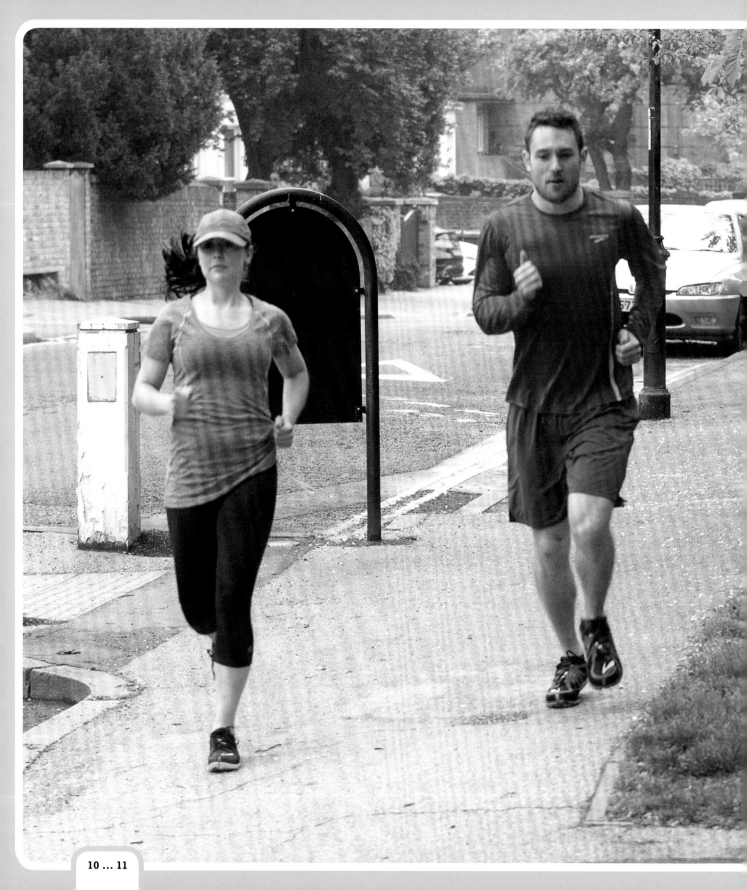

the road to the
revolution

that fitness didn't have to mean torture. Realising that getting breathless from rushing up the stairs to my bedroom at the age of 16 didn't bode well for the future, I decided I ought to force myself into some kind of exercise. I went to Woolworths and bought a Jane Fonda workout video, which was all the rage at the time (this was in the mid-1990s!). I gave it a go in the living room one day when the rest of the family weren't around and was astounded to find

> The calming sensation of physical tiredness was a revelation and I couldn't remember ever having slept so well. It also helped clear up my spotty teenage skin.

I quite enjoyed it. It wasn't easy, in fact, I found it incredibly tough, and had to pause the tape several times to catch my breath before re-joining Jane and her leg-warmer-clad aerobics class. (I still have no idea why woollen leg-warmers were considered necessary for sweaty indoor exercise classes back then.) But doing it felt good. It helped that I was on my own with no one there to snigger or shout at me for getting things wrong. The calming sensation of physical tiredness afterwards was a revelation too and I couldn't remember ever having slept so well. As a very pleasing bonus, it also seemed to help clear up my spotty teenage skin.

So, I kept at it and found I needed to pummel the pause button a little less every time. As the weeks went by I started to be able to move faster and noticed myself getting less malcoordinated. I found I had more energy and daily tasks that had previously been physically demanding, such as walking up the steep hill to my house, began to seem easy. Something was happening that I'd never experienced before: I was getting fitter.

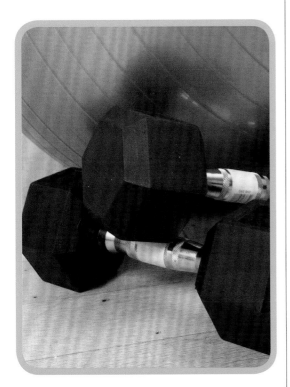

The only essential equipment is a set of dumbbells and an exercise ball.

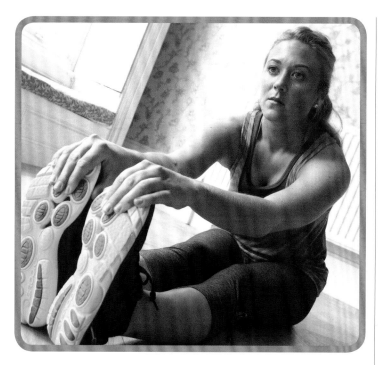

Confused by conflicting advice on the best type of exercise for fat loss? Read on and you'll learn why The Fat Burn Revolution is changing bodies and lives across the world.

Eventually I noticed I could match Jane and the leg-warmer-and-leotard crew in the advanced version of the workout. I could hardly believe I was doing it. Was I, Julia Buckley, now actually 'fit'?

I wondered if I might be capable of doing some other exercises that Jane hadn't shown me, maybe even alongside other people. So I did something I would never have imagined myself doing just a few months previously: I joined a gym.

Nearly 20 years later, I can still vividly remember what it felt like to be that young girl entering what was a very male-dominated environment in those days, whose only knowledge of exercise had been gleaned from a Jane Fonda video, trying to get to grips with the scary-looking equipment. It was daunting to say the least, but I enjoyed the challenge and was really excited about the changes I was noticing in my body and how I felt. I was also tremendously proud of myself to be even going to a gym. So I just kept going until, eventually, I started to become confident in that setting.

I've been a gym member ever since. I sometimes wonder how different my life and body would be today if I hadn't started out exercising in my parents' front room. Thanks, Jane!

A year or two later I got my first media job at a local radio station and my career in journalism began. Over the years I have worked for many high-profile media organisations and national titles (BBC, UKTV, *The Times*, the *Independent*, *Cosmopolitan*, *Closer*, to name a few). My passion for fitness has grown with every year and, looking back, it seems inevitable that I'd end up becoming a fitness writer (I've contributed to *Runner's World*, *WeightWatchers* magazine, *Bodyfit*, *Walk* magazine, *Trail Running*, and many more). Over the past few years I've also been taking on clients for personal training.

As a freelance fitness journalist, I am fortunate to

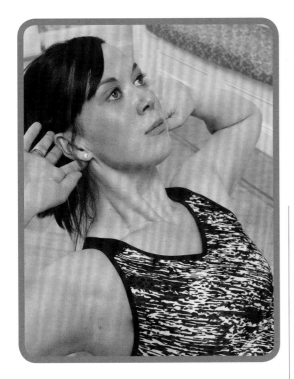

The training is intense, but the workouts are quite short and can all be done at home in your living room.

the **Fat Burn Revolution** is going to be a breeze for you, think again!

The **Fat Burn Revolution** is very adaptable and everyone is free to work at their own level – but for best results you should exercise at the very upper limits of those levels. You'll see what I mean once you've read more, but trust me, this is going to be a challenge whether you're already a regular exerciser or not.

If you don't feel fit, healthy and strong when you start the **Fat Burn Revolution**, you will by the end. And if you're already fit at the start, you'll be in sensational condition after 12 weeks!

If you don't feel fit, healthy and strong when you start the Fat Burn Revolution, you will by the end. And if you're already fit at the start, you'll be in sensational condition after 12 weeks!

As well as creating a programme that could be followed easily from home, I also wanted to introduce as many people as possible to the optimal type of training when losing fat is the main goal. I'll talk about the rationale behind the workouts and exercises later in the book, but be prepared for a programme that may be very different from the way you have exercised before.

have regular contact with many of the world's top sports scientists, coaches and fitness brands. I don't have allegiance to any particular company, publication or ethos, and this puts me in an excellent position to take an objective overview of what is going on in the world of fitness, and to see past over-hyped products, plans and gimmicks. I like to keep my focus on what really works for real people. I spend a lot of time on social media sites like Twitter, helping people to navigate their way through the fitness jungle! I do what I can, but I can only reach a certain group of people that way. So, after years of frustration about the mixed messages and conflicting and confused advice often conveyed in the media in relation to fat loss, not to mention scam 'secrets' promoted online, I decided it was time I created my own fat-loss fitness programme and shared it with the world.

One of my main priorities was that my programme should be beginner-friendly and accessible for anyone to do at home, with minimal equipment. However, if you're already in good shape and you're now thinking

getting you off the treadmill

I find it heart-breaking when I see the same people turn up to the gym week-in, week-out, month after month and year after year, sweating through long exercise sessions and trying their best to eat a good diet, but just not being able to shift the unwanted fat. Or there's the yo-yo exercisers who show up every January and/or just before their summer holidays, manage to scrape off a few pounds only to have gained it all back (plus extra) by the next time they squeeze through the gym turnstiles.

I promise you that it doesn't have to be that way, and it won't be for you once you understand the techniques and principles I'll be sharing with you in this book. Throughout the Fat Burn Revolution you will learn why exercise hasn't helped these people (maybe you're among them) to get lean. You'll also learn what you need to do to finally burn off that fat and get the body you want and deserve.

Before I discovered the fundamentals that the Fat Burn Revolution is based on, I used to push myself to all kinds of extremes to keep my fat levels under control and to feel like I was making progress in my fitness training. I spent excessive hours in the gym, attended ridiculous amounts of exercises classes (from aerobics to Zumba – you name it, I did it!) and I ran crazy amounts of miles (50-mile ultramarathon anyone?). I don't regret doing those things, and I (mostly) enjoyed it at the time (blisters, overuse injuries and overtraining-induced illnesses aside...).

Now I've experienced how much better I feel, how much better my body performs, how much my health has improved, and how much easier it is to maintain low levels of body fat by following this regime, I don't train that way any more.

But this is not about me; it's about you. I was sure that most people wanting to increase their fitness and lose fat would benefit from this programme, but before publishing a book on it, I wanted to get proof. So at the end of 2012 I put the word out online that I was looking for a group of people to test my 12-week fat-loss fitness programme. I gathered together a group of 20 people with a wide cross-section of backgrounds from across the UK, some with only a few pounds to lose, others with a few extra stones. Their circumstances ranged from busy mums to business owners to academics to fitness professionals. I was slightly concerned that I was taking a risk in gathering such a varied bunch, but I wanted to ensure that my methods would work for virtually anyone. The risk paid off.

I'm happy to report the results were even better than I had hoped. I was surprised and delighted and the participants were simply over the moon. I don't like using weight loss as a measure of the success of the Fat Burn Revolution because the numbers can be misleading, but people always ask, so, if we must talk weight, members of the group lost up to more than two stone in 12 weeks. Even more impressively, body-fat percentages fell by up to a massive 15%!

Here are some of their comments on the difference the Fat Burn Revolution programme made to them:

"

'I never would have dreamed I could lose 19 pounds in 12 weeks or that I would achieve such a change in body shape. It's so lovely now getting lots of positive compliments and feeling much better about myself. I still have more fat I'd like to lose, however I am much further down the line now than I anticipated. Now I know that I can do it I have more motivation to finally get the body I have always dreamed of.'

Kat, 26

'After not exercising for four years I was a bit worried about starting the programme, but I knew I had to make changes so I just went for it. I was surprised and pleased at how soon the changes started to happen. My body adapted to the exercises quickly and I didn't feel hungry following the eating guidelines – actually, I had to make an effort to ensure I ate enough to fuel my training. I learned so much during the programme and totally changed my thinking around exercise, there's no way I'm going back to being a couch potato again now!'

Simon, 41

'I got a hell of a lot out of those 12 weeks, I got rid of the stubborn fat from around my stomach, thighs and arms, and I also made some important changes to the way I thought about myself and my body. I now feel like I am armed with the toolbox to have an enjoyable and healthy future.'

Zoe, 37

'I'd thought I would probably drop one dress size, but not two! Being able to follow a smart schedule of workouts in the comfort of my own home, without the substantial on-going investment of joining a gym, knowing that Julia was only a message away to support me, gave me the flexibility I needed to fit exercise into my daily routine. Julia has encouraged me to aspire to a level of fitness that seemed unattainable just a few months ago.'

Sarah, 40

'As well as busting flab and boosting my fitness I have increased my flexibility and energy levels. The programme is inspiring and fun with punchy workouts that bring great results!'

Claire, 37

'After having both of my hips replaced I set myself the lofty goal of getting into the best shape of my life. Before I started this programme I would spend hours doing steady cardio workouts and became frustrated that my body shape wasn't changing. Julia convinced me to ditch that type in favour of short, hard fat burn and the results were magic!'

Alastair, 50

'I only wish I had known Julia 10 years ago post-babies. All those years of looking like a beached whale on holiday in swimwear! I've tried regular fitness classes, BMF, joining gyms, using PowerPlate, Insanity workout DVDs and more, but this programme is the most effective form of exercise I've ever done.'

Shelley, 42

'I dropped to a weight that I hadn't seen on the scales since I was child, but this time I didn't look like a scrawny little girl! I love having muscle definition, it makes me feel much more confident about my body.'

Vicki, 30

Please visit www.juliabuckley.co.uk to see some impressive before and after pictures.

2 get real, get results

The standard way to follow the Fat Burn Revolution is to exercise five to six days per week for twelve weeks, so that's what I'll assume you're going to do throughout the book. However, you are free to take things more gradually if you would prefer to work through the programme over a longer period of time. You will be using weights to sculpt your whole body and a stability ball to strengthen and firm up your core and tummy muscles. Plus you'll be sweating it out with fast-paced activity to super-charge your metabolism and accelerate your fitness.

Five to six days of training per week may be more frequent exercise than you might have seen recommended elsewhere, but I'd like you to forget that old 'three times per week is enough' advice. It's much better to get into the habit of making exercise a part of most of your days and, most importantly when shedding fat is your goal, daily exercise will keep your body burning lots of fat all the time, not just a few days per week. If time is an issue for you, don't worry, the workouts are challenging but they are short, some last less than 20 minutes, and all are less than an hour in duration.

> **You are going to be so glad you did this at the end of the 12 weeks. You will not regret a single ounce of the effort you put in.**

Ideally you will also do 15–30 minutes of low-intensity sustained exercise every day. This can be anything that gets you moving – walking, jogging, gardening, dancing, housework, swimming, shopping, playing with your child or dog, etc. You can choose any activity that will fit into your day for this element of the Fat Burn Revolution. This activity needs to be done at least six hours either before or after your workout of the day. So, if you do your workout in the morning, for example, you'll need to do your 15–30 minutes low-intensity session (say, taking the dog for a walk) in the evening, or vice versa.

The Fat Burn Revolution comprises three four-week phases and the workouts become more advanced as you progress. There will be no point at which the exercise becomes easy. If you find it easy, I don't care how fit or strong you are, you are doing it wrong! From total beginners to advanced exercisers,

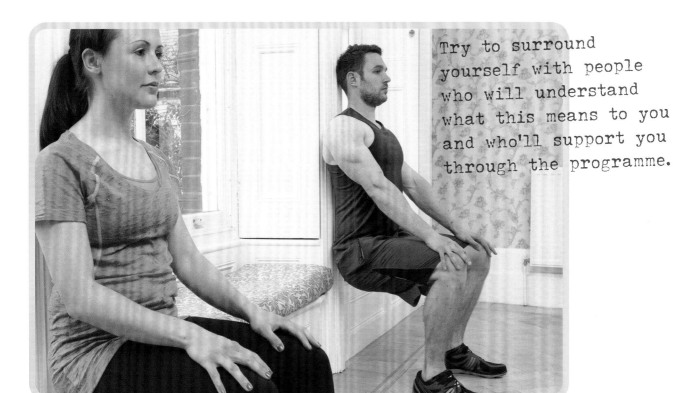

Try to surround yourself with people who will understand what this means to you and who'll support you through the programme.

we'll all be sweating together. Don't worry, though, you're not in for 12 weeks of hell, even people in the pilot group who previously hadn't exercised much before or had never liked working out with weights said they loved the workouts and I'm sure you'll find them enjoyable too. The feel-good factor of finishing one of these sessions is hard to match and you may well experience energy levels you've never known before by the end of the 12 weeks.

Of course, the changes you'll notice in the way your body looks, feels and performs will help keep you going too. Trust me, if you stick closely to the exercise schedule and dietary guidelines you will see improvement and you are going to be so glad you did by the end of 12 weeks. You will not regret a single ounce of the effort you put in.

If 12 weeks seems like a daunting amount of time to commit to rigorous daily exercise, I can tell you that those weeks are going to fly. It's worth noting

'I will neither deny nor make any apologies for the fact that this exercise schedule is tough. This is a real-world exercise programme that will get you real results. It is time for you to face up to the fact that to get the body you want you will have to work hard, push your limits and support your training with good eating habits.'

that one of the things many of the participants in the pilot group said in common at the end was that the 12 weeks seemed to go by in a flash. Many of them added that they'd wished they'd realised how quickly the time would pass in the early weeks when they felt they had time to catch up if they missed a few workouts or their eating went off course for a few days.

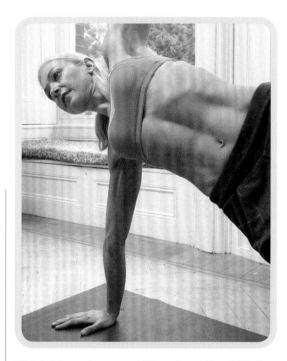

Think 12 weeks seems like a long time? Well, the time is going to pass anyway, so wouldn't you rather arrive at the end of it with an improved body?

That said, my advice is not to think in terms of 12 weeks stretching ahead, just take one day at a time. Simply take care of your 20–60 minute workout each training day and the weeks will take care of themselves.

I will explain the rationale behind the workouts, so you'll know why you're doing each of the exercises and the reasons they are part of your optimal fat-burning strategy. I want you to fully understand how this programme is going to work for you so you can really accept that it will absolutely get you the body you want if you follow it consistently.

It's important that you banish all doubts from your mind. I know this may be hard to do, especially if you have several failed attempts at fat loss under your belt (and who hasn't?). If you're cynical I don't blame you. With all the lies about various miraculous weight-loss products we're bombarded with nowadays, I totally understand that it is hard to believe a programme can be genuinely effective for ordinary people in the long term.

> The Fat Burn Revolution requires a very minimal outlay of time compared to the way the majority of people exercise, but it does require a substantial investment of effort. The returns, however, are spectacular.

But the fact is that fat loss is possible and it's something almost anyone can achieve if they take the correct action. To really get the most out of the Fat Burn Revolution you need to fully believe that and commit yourself 100 per cent to making it happen. Think about the people who helped test Fat Burn Revolution. These are real people – not celebrities or billionaires – they have jobs, kids and all the usual obligations and responsibilities that come with living in the real world. You heard from Kat (26) who dropped 19lbs and reduced her body-fat percentage from 31% to 24%; Shelly (42), the mum of three who, after just 12 weeks on the programme, finally got the flat belly she'd spent 10 years trying to achieve with various other forms of exercise; Simon (41) who lost 31lbs and discovered a new love of exercise; and more.

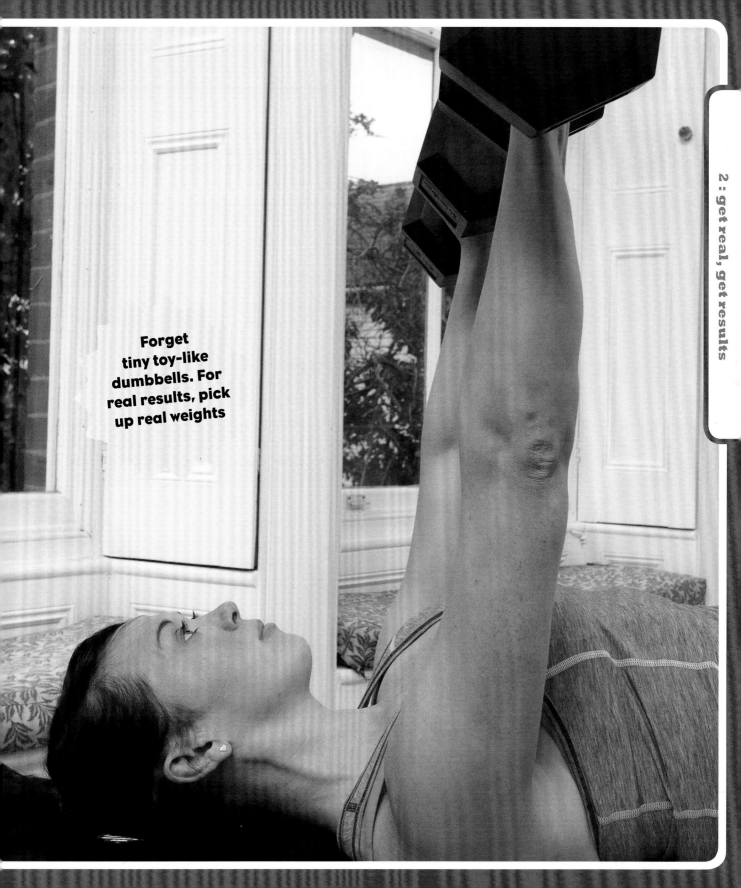

Forget tiny toy-like dumbbells. For real results, pick up real weights

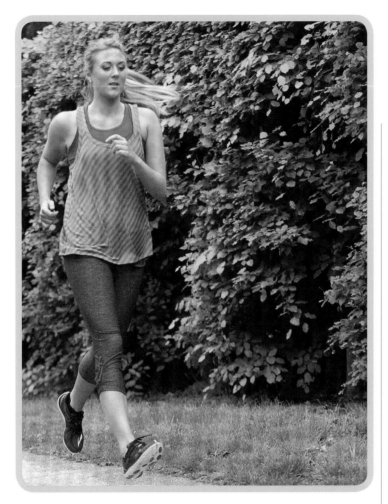

Many of the exercises activate muscles across the whole body to promote outstanding fat burning and fitness boosting results.

and get into amazing shape, simply follow the basic recommendations outlined in Chapter 5 to make sure you're putting the right foods into your body to get the best possible benefits and results.

Following the programme will not only be a physical challenge, you will need to stay mentally focused and dedicated to honouring the commitment you have made to yourself to see this through. I'll give you as much help, advice and inspiration as I can through my words in this book and online support materials, but ultimately it is down to you to put everything into practice and make the results happen.

The journey you are about to take will almost certainly change you as a person. As a result, you will find the benefits of following this programme extend beyond the physical. The change might be very subtle or it could be quite dramatic, but you won't be quite the same person upon finishing the Fat Burn Revolution as you were at the start. You'll be stronger and more resilient, mentally as well as physically, you'll become more self-motivated, ready to rise to challenges or try new things, and you'll be more confident in yourself as a person, as well as in relation to your body. It's life-changing stuff we're talking about here!

Of course, you won't have forgotten who you were just 12 weeks before. You'll be well aware that, like most people, you have the propensity to gain fat and, let's face it, be lazy. But at the same

As well as giving everything you've got in the exercise sessions, to get the body you want chances are you will need to make changes to the way you eat. Most 'diets' work, at least in the short term and if you are already following an eating plan, which is working for you and you want to continue with that alongside the Fat Burn Revolution fitness programme, that's fine. Or, you can follow my recommendations, which are the same guidelines that helped the pilot group shed fat time as shedding fat you are going to be gaining willpower, confidence and self-motivation, which will be reflected in all areas of your life. This will happen gradually, bit by bit. You probably won't even notice it at first, but by the end you'll be aware that something feels different inside. You will have become someone who gets up and takes the necessary action whether you feel energetic, motivated and inspired, or not.

The deeper you embed your healthy habits by repeating them consistently, the easier it will be to stay on course in the long term and, should you ever waiver off-course, the clearer your road map back to fitness will be. I said in Chapter 1 that you should not expect the training to ease once you have 'mastered' the programme, because that won't happen. However, as the weeks go by you will find that getting yourself to do the training will become less of struggle. There are many reasons for this. For a start you'll be fitter and more energetic, plus seeing your new body shape emerge is going to get you really excited about continuing. But perhaps the main thing that's going to make lacing up your training shoes feel like a natural part of your day is that it will have simply become part of your normal routine. Once you've got into the habit of doing the workouts and your mind starts to realise that it's a non-negotiable part of your day, you won't hear half so much whingeing and excuse-making from that whiny voice in your head that doesn't want you to

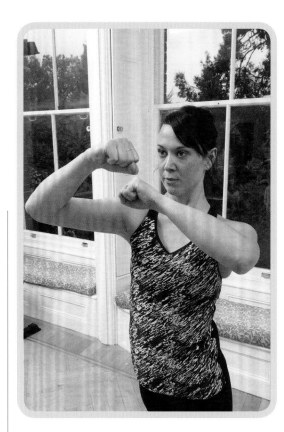

ever achieve anything so that it can complain even more. That voice might pipe up a lot during the first few weeks, by the way. But that's OK, just exercise anyway. The more you ignore it, the quieter it'll get.

Motivation and willpower come and go in waves for even the keenest among us and sometimes there are days when even having established good habits isn't enough to get us off our backsides. However, there is one thing that can absolutely guarantee your success if only you choose to embrace it. That is commitment, and we will be looking at that in more detail in the next chapter.

> I can only give you the map, it's you who has to make the journey.

3 commit to the cause

To give yourself the best chances of getting the best possible results, before you begin the Fat Burn Revolution you should get clear in your own mind what you want to achieve over the next 12 weeks and the reasons why. For example, do you want to look better in your clothes? To look better out of them? To have more energy? More confidence? To feel stronger mentally and/or physically? To put habits into place that will help you stay healthy and mobile into your senior years? The possible benefits are endless, but which are most important to you?

> 'The road to success is paved with commitment. If you don't have commitment under your feet, no matter how much you want to be at your destination, you're not going to get there.'

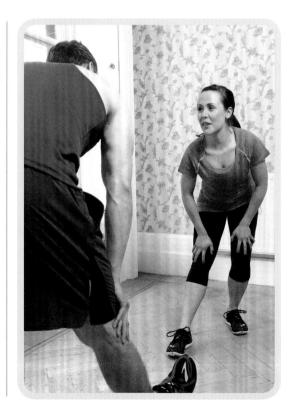

Make a list of at least 20 ways in which getting into shape and shedding fat will make your life better. Once you have that list, put it somewhere you'll see it regularly – ideally on the fridge door to remind you of what making a poor food choice could cost you. Try to memorise the list and repeat it to yourself when you have an idle few minutes to think, such as on your commute to work or waiting on hold on the phone. Add more reasons whenever they come to mind and remind yourself of them if you find your motivation starting to wane.

seek out support

I highly recommend you seek out someone, or a group of people, to be support buddies who will keep an eye on your progress, and you can do them same for them if they are also looking to become more physically fit. Approach people who you know will be supportive and positive, but won't let you get away with excuses. Explain to them what the Fat Burn Revolution is all about and what it means to you to see this through. Send or show them your journal regularly (ideally once a week. See page 189) throughout the programme and talk to them about the progress you're making and how that makes you feel.

If you don't have anyone suitable in your life, no problem, you can join the incredibly supportive group of people who are currently following, or have previously completed, the Fat Burn Revolution via juliabuckley.co.uk.

Most of us are much better at sticking to our plans when we know someone else is watching. Even if you're super-self-motivated, it's always nice to get a bit of encouragement from other people. Having at least one person you know will be right behind you throughout the next 12 weeks could really help keep you on track because unfortunately, it's likely you will find that not everyone in your life will be supportive of you all of the time.

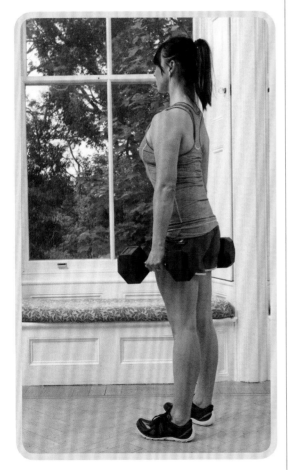

One of the many benefits you may experience from following this programme is improved posture, which will improve your silhouette, make you look more confident and protect your back.

> Reading about other people's experiences is a great way to get inspiration and reassurance, visit juliabuckley.co.uk to join the community of others following this programme. I'll be adding more resources to the site all the time, so look out for even more helpful features coming soon.

friendly fire

When a person makes changes to the way they live their life it usually takes a while for the people around them to get used to the idea. Even though eating a more nutritious diet and exercising regularly are very positive changes you may well come up against resistance from the people around you.

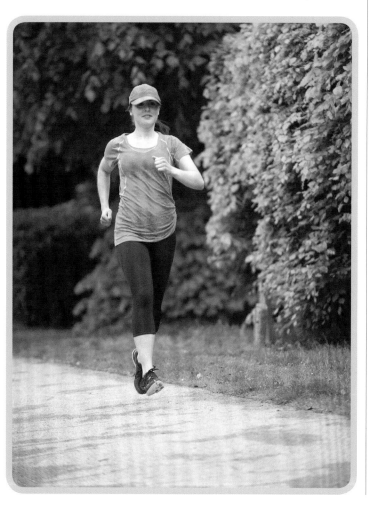

Problems can range from people trying to tempt you with your favourite sugar-loaded snacks or trying to persuade you to join them in a booze-up, to attempting to make you feel guilty for taking time out to exercise, to disputing your need to make changes, even to trying to discourage you by saying you're unlikely to succeed.

You certainly wouldn't be the first to come up against all of that and more. I hear about it all of the time. People are often shocked by the opposition they face from people who they thought would totally understand that they've had enough of being dragged down by excess body fat.

The problem is other people haven't been riding your train of thought, they don't know about all the agonising that's been going on in your head.

A lot of people simply don't like change, especially in other people. They are usually scared of what it might mean, they like you just fine the way you are after all. Which is nice. But it's not them who has to live with your flab on their body is it?

Sometimes their motives will be complex, possibly to do with their own body issues or personal insecurities. Maybe they have their own excess fat to contend with, and maybe that's part of the reason why seeing you set off on a fat-busting mission is upsetting to them. Or they might simply not realise that their behaviour is making it difficult for you to stick to a plan that is going to improve your life. With time they'll get used to the new you and when they see the fantastic difference the changes make to you, they may even join you.

how to deal with unsupportive people

get real

Yes, it would be lovely if everyone around you was wonderfully supportive and applauded all your fitness training, never offered you any fattening food and gave you tons of encouragement. But that's not what tends to happen in real life, so it's not what you should expect to get.

Expect people to try to tempt you with poor food choices. Anticipate that they will try to talk you into doing other things during your exercise time. Presume that sometimes people will attempt to make you feel guilty about the changes you're making. When you know that's how it's going to be, you can plan how to deal with it.

share your reasons

Explain in as much detail and with as much enthusiasm as you can muster what getting leaner and healthier means to you. Go through your list of reasons why you're following the Fat Burn Revolution and talk about how it has already made you feel better. Let them know you would value their support and lay out in very simple terms what they can do to be supportive. Things that may seem obvious to you may not be so apparent to them, so spell it out. Even if it makes no difference, at least you'll know you tried.

own it

Always remember that it is totally up to you what you eat. You are an adult and no one can make you eat or drink anything you don't want to. Your body is entirely your own and if you want to exercise to get it into better condition you should feel completely free to go ahead and do that.

Making healthy lifestyle changes in the midst of unsupportive people can be tough, but sticking to the Fat Burn Revolution despite objectors is great training to build up strong 'willpower muscles' that will help keep you on course through the inevitable ups and downs life will throw at you.

be direct

Make your healthy choices and don't invite unhelpful comments from others by intimating that you'd rather be doing anything else. If someone offers you something to eat or drink that you don't want, turn it down politely, but not apologetically. Say something like, 'No, thanks' or 'Thanks, but I'm not hungry.' Do not say things like, 'Oh I really shouldn't' or 'I can't I'm on a diet.' Because what do you think their reaction is going to be if you say the latter? Even if the food does look tempting, you don't have to say it out loud. Use the same principle if someone tries to talk you out of exercising with offers of doing something else instead.

it's about you

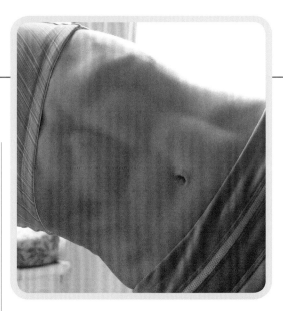

Dreaming of a flat stomach? I will show you how to make it a reality if you consistently put my advice into action.

Support is great when you can get it, but always remember that you, and you alone, are the only person who can take action to achieve the fat loss you want.

Hopefully I've said enough to convince you that the Fat Burn Revolution will get you leaner, fitter and healthier. But, as I mentioned, the programme is just a map, it is down to you to make a firm commitment to follow it.

Everyone would like to have a great body, but not many people are ready to make the commitment and take the consistent daily action it takes to get into shape. But get your mind in the right place and you will make it happen.

Before you start punching the air declaring your absolute commitment to the Fat Burn Revolution, let's have a quick look at what commitment really means.

Some people set goals and then simply sit around fantasising about how great it will be once they've achieved them. That is definitely not what commitment is. Commitment is about getting the job done. I want you to get excited about the results you will achieve, but I also want you to be in no doubt that if you do not do the workouts and if you do not support those workouts with a healthy diet,

you will not get those results. The fat will absolutely stay on your body and in all likelihood continue to expand if you don't take action. You have to take action, repeatedly and consistently. Don't ever let fantasising about how wonderful it's going to be when you reach your goal distract you from what you need to do in order to get there.

One of the reasons I urge you to take Before photos at the beginning of the programme is to help you to enforce that commitment. At times when you feel like missing a workout or are about to make a poor food choice I want you to look at that photo and remind yourself of the reality and the commitment you've made to change. You are not going to get the body you want by wishing for it really hard, or imagining it really vividly, or by sitting around thinking how wonderful everything's going to be once you've got it. You are going to it get by consistently making good choices and taking action – on days when you feel like it and on days when you don't.

 If you decide now that quitting is not an option, you won't eliminate all the bumps in the road, but you will reach your goal in the end.

dream on

Contrary to what you may have read in self-help books, new research shows that regularly picturing yourself achieving your dreams could actually make you less likely to achieve them. People who do this tend to crumble when they hit obstacles because they are not mentally prepared for the effort and determination they need in order to get the results they want.

When you think about it, it is simple human nature to expect things to be easier than they end up being. We all do it. How many times have you misjudged how quickly you could get a project done, or been late for something because getting there took longer than you expected? Everyone falls into the same trap, all the time. Shedding fat and getting into shape is definitely no exception.

However, your imagination can still play a part in helping you achieve fat loss through the use of visualisation techniques.

visualisation techniques

Visualisation techniques have become an established element of sports psychology. There is a lot of evidence to show that athletes who vividly imagine themselves putting in outstanding performances are more likely to achieve the result they want. (Visualisation is also used in addiction therapy, where people imagine themselves dealing with situations where they would previously have indulged their addiction.)

What sportspeople are doing is visualising the process of achieving their goals rather than focusing only on the end results. They are not kidding themselves that they've already got there, but getting their minds mentally prepared to do what needs to be done.

Think about the aspects of following the programme that are likely to present the biggest challenges for you. Will it be turning down offers of fattening foods? Not snacking on processed junk? Getting out of bed and exercising early in the morning? Or when you arrive home from work tired and hungry?

Think carefully about what issues will arise, then make a plan and in your mind's eye visualise yourself dealing with them. If you feel anxious during this process, that's a sign that you need to do it all the more, so stick with those feelings and work through them by showing yourself how you'll tackle those testing situations.

The very fact that you're reading this book is proof that you have had enough of settling for less than the best you can be and you are ready to take action to improve your life. Obstacles will come up along the way, some of which you may not foresee right now, but there will always be a way of dealing with them and moving towards your goal. Of course, doubts will appear, and you will have lazy days when you'd rather be doing anything but your scheduled workout. But you've now committed to success, so you'll do it anyway. And you will not regret it.

4 metabolic magic

Occasionally I might use the vernacular and talk about 'weight loss', because it helps me get my message out into the mainstream, but really what happens to people on the Fat Burn Revolution programme is that they shed fat and gain muscle and become leaner, fitter and their bodies look hotter as a result.

Although not a pretty picture, try searching for images of five pounds of body fat and five pounds of muscle on the internet. I'm asking you to do this to realise that a person's weight may not tell the full story when they make changes to their body shape. Take a good look at the pictures and ask yourself, which would look better on my thighs or arms? As you can see, if you removed five pounds of fat from your body and gained five pounds of muscle you would look a lot smaller, while the scales would not move. This is a principle I really want you to understand before you start your Fat Burn Revolution journey.

I do suggest that you record your weight, but the main reason for this is to help you see that the plan is 'working' and that you are indeed losing fat.

> When all is said and done, who really cares what they weigh? I know I don't! It's how we look and feel and how healthy we are that counts.

But be aware that changes in weight do not always show you what is really happening to your body. The scales can be distorted by hydration levels, the amount of food in your system, hormonal cycles (which affect both men and women) and many other factors. Typically, people will experience losing a lot of weight in the first two or three weeks of any diet and/or exercise programme and then the weight loss will slow down, which can be demotivating. (Don't be fooled by TV weight loss shows, by the way, they deliberately select severely obese participants so those big drops will continue for longer, but I'll restrain myself from ranting about that here.) However, it's not all bad. Often this initial weight loss helps people finally make the connection between the shape of their body and the food and exercise choices they've been making. At last, they see there is no mystery to it. They don't need to wait around in vain for a magical weight-loss pill to be invented or accept that they have no choice but to always be weighed down by excess fat. The fact that they have lost weight gives them the proof they need to see that they can control the amount of

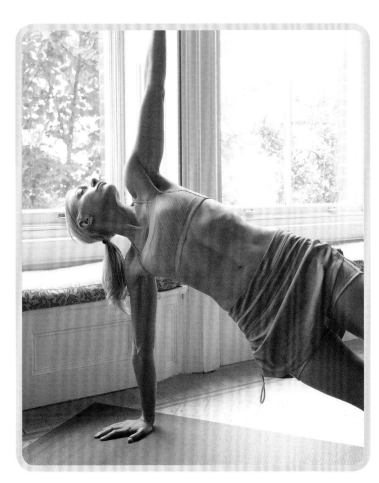

For just 12 weeks, let go of:
- Excuses
- Procrastination
- Sitting and hoping
- Negativity and self-doubt
- Laziness
- Mindless eating/drinking
- Fear of failure

...And anything else that has held you back in the past. When you see the difference this makes, you won't want them back.

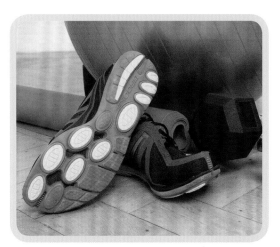

fat stored in their bodies by doing the right kind of exercise and eating the right kinds of foods.

In an ideal world, we'd just look in the mirror or notice how our clothes felt to gauge progress. Unfortunately, for the vast majority of us, our perceptions of our bodies are too distorted for that. Most of us find it difficult to notice when we're getting fatter and the same goes when we're getting leaner. But when you see the numbers get lower on the scale or measuring tape, then you have the evidence that proves fat loss is happening and that what you're doing is causing changes to occur. It is very possible to have a lean sculpted physique and weigh a lot more than someone whose body looks overweight and out of shape. So please don't get hung up on those numbers.

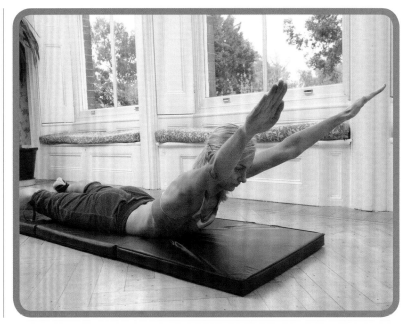

the miracle of muscle

As well as taking a Before photo, I highly recommend you take progress photos every three or four weeks and compare them to your Before shots. You should now realise that the Fat Burn Revolution is not a diet plan, what you are doing is creating a great body shape at the same time as gradually shedding fat. As you strip back that fat, what will be revealed is a firm, fit-looking physique that you can happily maintain in the long term.

Adding muscle not only gives your body a firmer, more attractive shape, it improves athletic performance, reduces injury risk, aids mobility and agility, reduces aches and pains, brings a huge range of health benefits and, of course, makes you stronger. And, as I've said in previous chapters, beyond the physical, all of this transfers into increased confidence and general well-being.

All that aside, the benefit of the Fat Burn Revolution that many people get most excited about is the fact that adding muscle to the body increases the metabolic rate.

Metabolic rate is a measurement of the amount of fuel your body uses. The problem with most weight-loss diet and exercise programmes is that they actually reduce metabolic rate. Believe it or not, the fat you have on your body places an extra demand on your daily energy requirements just by being there, as it needs to be maintained. So, when you shed flab, the amount of fuel you burn each day will fall. If you ate the same diet you did before without increasing your activity levels, even if that diet had previously been just right – neither causing you to gain or lose weight – you will now be putting more fuel into your body than it needs and the excess will be stored as fat. Obviously, to lose additional fat you then have to keep eating less and less or exercising more and more.

I'm afraid it gets worse. Following most weight-loss diet and exercise plans will also cause muscle to be lost from your body along with the fat. Muscle requires even more energy to maintain on the body than fat but it is much smaller and smoother than fat (weight for weight), so a reduction in this type of tissue can be disastrous for your body shape.

If you restrict calories and either don't exercise or choose traditional forms of cardiovascular 'weight-loss' exercise (like steady-paced aerobics, running or cycling), while you may lose weight in the short term, in the process you will probably lose muscle and slow down your metabolism. This means that once you go back to your normal lifestyle it will be very difficult to maintain your results and even more difficult to lose weight in the future. Yep, it's a bummer!

Muscles
burn fat

If you've got your head around this, you'll now see how the majority of people who lose weight tend to eventually regain even more fat than they started with.

You should also be starting to realise why, for most people, adding muscle to the body should be an essential aspect of their fat-loss attack plan. Hopefully now you also fully understand why it is not a good idea for you to measure your progress on this programme by weight alone.

> A lot of women tend to store more fat on their lower halves, but when they strip back the fat it reveals a gorgeous shapely pair of pins.

will you turn into Popeye?

If you're concerned that gaining muscle will make you look too big and bulky, please put that out of your head. This is something that tends to worry women more than men, but ladies, I can assure you that getting big muscles is very hard for us to achieve even when we try to. It definitely does not happen by accident when we're not specifically training for that aim. Guys do get that 'ripped' look they usually want by following the Fat Burn Revolution because their bodies produce more testosterone and they gain muscle more easily. Women, on the other hand, get lean, firm and shapely.

I'm not saying anything sexist or controversial here, by the way, these are just simple biological facts. If you're old enough to be reading this I'm sure you've noticed that male and female bodies are different! So it shouldn't be all that shocking to hear that both sexes can follow the same programme, but men's bodies will react to it differently by increasing muscle size at a greater rate than a woman's body will.

Successful female bodybuilders usually do an astounding amount of training and follow a very strict diet, usually involving periods of eating a large quantities of calories during carefully planned muscle-building phases and regularly swallowing a range of supplements. What I'm basically saying is that women who train and eat to get bulky do not do what you will do while following the Fat Burn Revolution.

Another common concern I've come across, again usually among women, is not wanting to use weights in leg exercises because they think they already have 'bulky' legs. In fact, what they've almost always actually got is fat sitting on top of muscle. They find it hard to accept that it's fat because it looks and even feels like it's all muscle, but it is not. Believe me, I've seen this many times on many women, including myself.

I put weight on a while ago when I had a calf injury and I went to see a physiotherapist who looked at my leg using an ultrasound scanner. I was really surprised when I looked at the screen and could see quite a thick layer of fat on top of the muscle. My calves had felt quite hard, so I didn't think I had much fat in that area, but there it was. When I lost the fat (with weighted leg exercises as part of my training) my calves shrank and I'm very happy with the shape of them now.

say goodbye to your comfort zone

If you've been exercising for a while, chances are you've experienced reaching a progress plateau. This frustrating phenomenon has been the cause of many an abandoned fitness goal. It is also the reason why going to the same exercise class or following the same routine for months on end does not tend to get people the body they want. Training consistency is a wonderful thing, but never changing the way you train is not.

Typically it goes like this. You decide to start a new fitness regime and find a workout/class/DVD you like the look of. At first it's great, the fat starts coming off and it seems like you've found 'The Answer'. After a few weeks you start getting used to the moves, it all feels a lot easier, and doing the workout begins to feel comfortable. So, great, you're getting fitter, right? But here's the thing, pretty soon you start to notice that it isn't shifting any more. You probably don't worry much about that at first, after all, you know this training works, so you resolve to keep going and stick with it. However, the weeks go by and still nothing changes and doing the same routine starts getting boring, especially as you're not being rewarded with any results. So, your willpower starts to wane and you lose interest. Who could blame you when nothing is changing? Before long the sofa becomes a much a more appealing option and, after several missed weeks, workout time becomes TV time and eventually you don't even think about exercising any more. Sound familiar?

Let's move on from that depressing scenario. I have good news. Can you guess what it is?

Yep, that sequence of events is not a problem

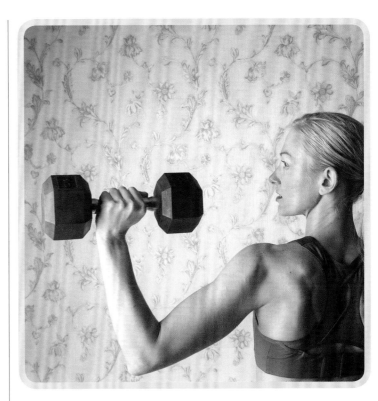

Your workout schedule will change every 4 weeks, so your body will be constantly challenged throughout the programme.

you'll have on the Fat Burn Revolution programme. There may be occasional weeks when you don't lose weight, or even any body fat, but there will always be a way to increase the intensity to ensure your progress is not stalled for long. Plus, by changing the workouts every four weeks, your body will not be given time to get comfortable with the demands you're placing on it. Remember what I said about continually challenging yourself and it never getting easy? You'll thank me for it after 12 weeks!

running into trouble

I know I'm labouring the point a little now, but I really want to embed this message in the very depths of your being: comfortable workouts are not going to get you the results you want. I've already mentioned the muscle-reducing dangers of endurance-type exercise like leisurely running, cycling or swimming, but there's more.

Before I go on, I want to stress that I have nothing against these types of exercise, I enjoy them all myself, I have completed several marathons and even used to be the editor of a magazine for recreational runners. But the fact is that steady-paced running is not great for fat loss.

The typical story is similar to the sorry tale above and, unfortunately, the ending is often even sadder. It goes like this:

1 You take up running and you shed some weight and get fitter. Woohoo!

2 After a few weeks or, if you're lucky, months, the results slow down as you reach a plateau.

3 So, you decide to push yourself more, maybe to complete a race, after all it's good to have training goals, everyone knows that. You increase your training time and up your mileage.

4 You see some more gains, but these plateau out even more quickly. Your body, being the wonderful machine that it is, just keeps adapting to cope with the strain.

5 It's not easy to fit in more training and increased mileage, but you're not going to quit, it's all about pushing through the pain, right?

6 And so you carry until you eventually have to stop because your body can't take it any more and you get ill or injured.

7 You are forced to stop training and you gain even more fat.

Fun times eh?

Believe me, I've been there myself so I know how frustrating and confusing that cycle can be.

Any type of long, slow-endurance exercise, when done regularly and taken to extremes, will cause the body to become more endurance-focused. It will then want to store energy as fat to ensure it has plenty of reserves to get through all the miles it is expecting and it will release those fat stores very sparingly.

Unfortunately, the problems don't end there. Endurance sports involve such repetitive movements that, unless you have perfect biomechanics (i.e. you have faultless posture and gait), which almost nobody does, the more miles you do and the more often you train, the more likely it becomes that those imbalances and imperfections in your gait are going to lead to pain and injury. Even if that doesn't happen you're at risk of general overuse injuries and then there's the damaging effects excessive endurance training may have on the heart and endocrine system... I think you're getting the point now!

Running, cycling and swimming can be fantastic in small amounts, but many people (including me) get carried away and keep upping their mileage without realising that their training is at odds with their health/fitness/fat-loss goals.

enter the Revolution

When you train using high-intensity cardio, plyometrics and challenging resistance sessions, as in the Fat Burn Revolution, the body prefers to store fuel as glycogen in the muscles. This type of fuel can be

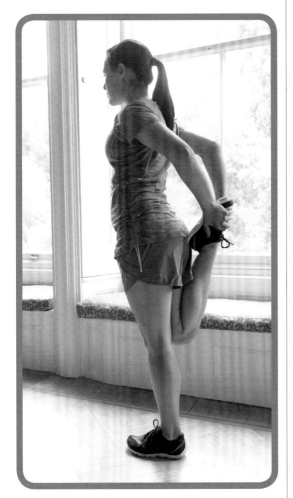

The intense training will prime your body to burn off fat stores long after you've finished exercising.

quickly released to enable the fast-paced, power-driven activities it is used to performing.

How will this get rid of the fat on your body? Because of the 'afterburn' effect. You are going to train so hard your metabolic rate will go through the roof and it will stay high even after you finish training while your body adapts and recovers. This will cause you to burn more fat for 24–48 hours after exercising, depending on how intense the training was. Of course, you also get the health and fitness improvements that come as a result of working your heart, lungs and muscles harder.

You may have been told that exercising at a comfortable pace is best for fat loss because you are working in the 'fat-burning zone'. This is just plain wrong. People who say this are confused by the fact that training at low intensities causes the body to use more fat than glycogen for fuel while you are exercising. But what they don't realise is that high-intensity exercise causes more fat to be burned in total when you take account of afterburn. Plus, with this type of training, the next time you eat, the calories from your food will be used to replace the glycogen you used up rather than stored as fat.

By following the Fat Burn Revolution you will shed more fat, experience fewer injuries, improve your health, get a better body shape, increase your energy levels and with your accelerated metabolism it will be easier to maintain your leaner physique in the long term. Plus, as bonus, you won't need to spend as much time exercising.

If deciding to switch to this type of training now sounds like a no-brainer, that's because it is.

5 you wear what you eat

If you want a great body, you're going to have to eat a great diet.

The Fat Burn Revolution workouts will burn off the fat stored on your body due to your past habits of eating the wrong foods and not doing the right kind of exercise. But if you continue to eat that way now, you will simply keep replacing those fat stores and you won't get the results you want.

I know this is going to sound simplistic but, when it comes down to it, it is as clear cut as this: you have to accept that the reason the excess fat is on your body is because you have been taking in, via food and drinks, more fuel than your body needs so that your body has cleverly stored it as fat to use up later. Don't worry, starting the Fat Burn Revolution will give your body the signal that 'later' has arrived and it's time to dip into those fat stores, but it will only work effectively once you stop overfeeding yourself.

If you're hoping to find a way around that truth, forget it, there isn't one. If you want a better body, you're going to have to make changes to what you eat. I'm asking you now: what would you rather have, fantastic physical fitness, huge reserves of energy

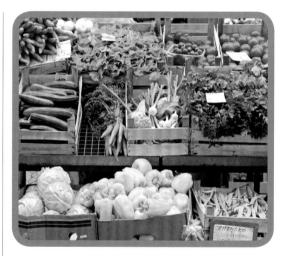

The days of guiltily cramming tasteless, cheap foods into your mouth are over. Nourish your body and it will thrive.

 When people make the changes I'm about to recommend they usually enjoy their food and feel more satisfied after eating than they did before.

and a strong sexy body, or to eat lots of processed foods that make you feel like crap? The choice is yours, but it sounds like another no-brainer to me!

The good news is that you don't have to starve yourself. In fact, you don't even need to give up eating any type of food entirely.

cancel calorie-counting and ditch the diet

As you learned in the previous chapter, the Fat Burn Revolution is going to put your body in a state where you burn fat around the clock, so it's not necessary to start trying to calculate how many calories you torched during sessions in order to allow yourself a related amount of food.

In my experience, people do best when they abandon the calorie-counting mentality. It's good to know which foods are calorie-dense and which aren't, but that is not the only aspect foods should be judged on, and daily calorie allowances are not the best way to manage your diet while following this programme.

Don't think of the changes you're going to make to what you eat as going 'on a diet'. You are going to be making long-term changes to the way you eat that you can maintain for life. There is no structured daily meal plan or recipe book alongside the Fat Burn Revolution book. This programme is for adults. You are a grown-up and you can decide for yourself what meals you're going to eat. You may be wishing I'd make it simpler for you by telling you exactly what to eat and when, but in the long run you're going to be a lot better off by learning to choose and prepare nourishing foods that fit your tastes and lifestyle.

So, you are free to eat whatever you like. I am simply going to offer you some advice in the form of the following guidelines. These guidelines are simple and flexible, but incredibly effective for reducing body fat, improving energy levels and generally ensuring your body gets what it needs to thrive.

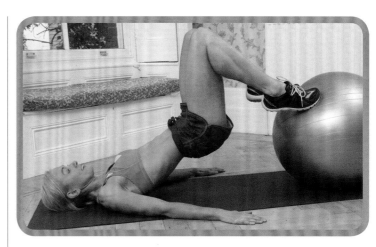

By now you should be starting to understand why, when fat burning is the main aim, this type of training is the way to go.

Sugar addicted? Hang in there: the cravings for overly sweet foods will pass as you begin to beat the addiction.

eliminate sugar No surprises here. Processed sugar offers virtually no nutritional value to your body, it plays havoc with your hormones and ultimately puts the body into fat-storing mode. You may get a momentary sugar rush right after eating it, but you start to feel hungry and tired very soon afterwards. For a lot of people, this is also accompanied by feelings of guilt and gloom, which last far longer than the few seconds the sweet taste lingered in their mouths. In short, sugar is really not worth eating and should be avoided wherever

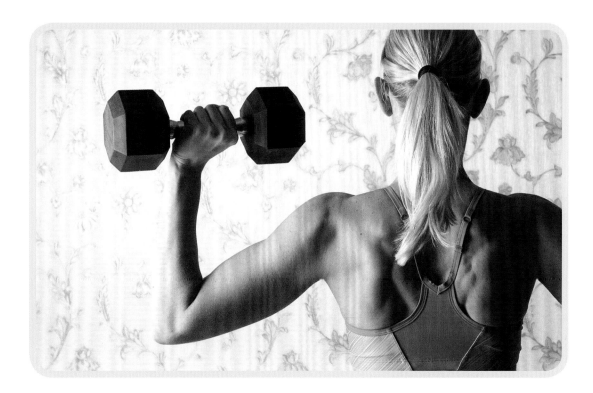

possible while fat loss is your priority. It is also horribly addictive, as you will probably realise as you begin to remove it from your diet.

replace grains and cereals with vegetables   Cereals, rice, bread, pasta and other foods made with flour, like pastry, are poor food choices. These are full of the 'empty' carbohydrates that caused you to store excess fat on your body. Plus they make you feel tired and bloated. These foods offer very few useful nutrients and are almost as bad for you as sugar. Keep reminding yourself these foods are tasteless, cheap bulk, which your body doesn't need or respond well too. You deserve better. Replace them whenever you can with lovely nutrient-rich vegetables, which will nourish and energise you.

do not drink your calories   Avoid calorie-laden beverages. Apart from the fact that they usually contain all kinds of nasty ingredients, they do not satisfy you the way food does. When your aim is to shed fat, it is much better to get your energy from food. Even smoothies and juice drinks are generally not good choices. It is much better to eat fruits and vegetables than grind them up and drink them. By eating them you benefit from the fibre contained in the pulp, which slows down the rate at which the carbohydrates are absorbed by the body and also makes you feel full and satisfied.

eat lean protein at every meal
Protein-rich foods are usually very tasty and they help you to feel 'full' and satisfied. Protein is also important for supporting the body as it adapts to the demands of the exercises in this programme. Getting enough of this nutrient in your diet is essential to ensure your body will perform at its best and recover quickly between sessions. Great choices include oily fish, lean cuts of meat, eggs, and Quorn products.

Eat protein-rich foods to build fat-burning, body sculpting muscle.

limit dairy products Milk is pretty disgusting when you think about what it is. Most people would find the idea of putting human breast milk on their cereal in the morning revolting, so how come we don't feel the same about the lactate of another species? Surely that should be even more disgusting – at least human milk is meant for baby humans rather than baby cows! I'm not saying you should limit your consumption of milk purely for squeamish reasons though, but mainly because of all the growth hormones and lactose (milk sugar) it contains, which will inhibit your fat loss. By all means have splash of milk in hot drinks if you like, but try to keep it to a minimum.

go easy on the booze A large glass of beer or wine could well contain the same amount of calories as a piece of cake or a chocolate bar. Yet a lot of people who wouldn't dream of eating three or four chocolate bars in one sitting regularly down that number of alcoholic drinks in an evening. When you take a tipple, don't think that because you're not eating the calories they won't impede your fat loss. Learn to think of alcohol in the same way as you're going to think of cake or chocolate: a small amount occasionally is OK, but several servings on a daily basis will absolutely keep you fat.

drink water and green tea Being in a dehydrated condition saps your energy, makes you think you're hungry when you aren't and generally makes you feel like crap. So drink lots of water. Have at least one glass with every meal. This will help you to feel fuller sooner and aid the digestion of your food. I'm a big fan of green tea, it's great for weight loss because it curbs cravings, suppresses appetite and there is some compelling scientific evidence that it boosts fat burning.

get your timing right You should refuel with a good meal as soon as you can after the workouts in this programme to get the maximum benefits and ensure you recover well so that you're ready for your next session. Opinions vary on whether to eat before exercise, so you may want to experiment to discover what works best for you. However, you should try to avoid timing a big meal immediately before a workout because there is a chance you will get stomach aches/cramps or sickness. There's a lot of evidence to suggest that eating late at night is detrimental to fat loss, and it can disturb sleep, so avoid this. Brush your teeth, go to bed and look forward to a good breakfast in the morning.

always think before you eat Before you put any food inside your mouth consider how you'll feel after you eat it, not just while you're eating it. And ask yourself if you are really hungry. If you are truly hungry you'll happily chomp through a plate of, say, fish, green beans, carrots and peas. If all you want to eat is a doughnut or bag of crisps, then what you are experiencing is not real hunger. It's most likely that it's your sugar/carb addiction rearing its ugly head. Ignore it and it'll pass. The more times you ignore it, the easier it will get and the less often it will happen.

if you are truly hungry, eat There's no need to go hungry, just don't reach for processed carbohydrates or sugary foods. Always keep nutritious foods on hand to chomp on when you need them. If you let yourself get too hungry your insulin levels will drop and your cravings for sugars and carbs will get worse, so do yourself a favour and fill up on good nourishing foods before hunger levels get too high.

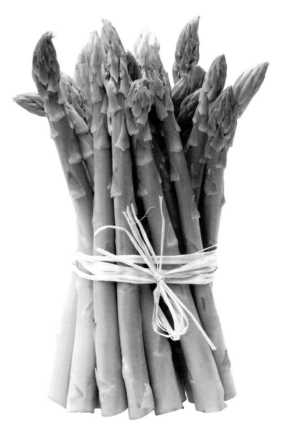

Think carefully before deciding what foods to eat, you'll be wearing the consequences later.

mostly healthy, most of the time

I want to stress that these are not 'rules' that you have to stick rigidly to 100% of the time. A daily slice of wholemeal bread, small portion of brown rice, the odd dessert or even an occasional 'cheat meal' won't thwart your Fat Burn Revolution.

My personal mantra is, 'Mostly healthy, most of the time'. What I mean by this is that it is what you habitually eat that determines how much fat is on your body, rather than what you eat very occasionally. So just make sure that the majority of the food you put into your body is healthy and nutritious and you should be able to get away with the odd less wholesome bite!

Most people who are overweight in the Western world got that way by filling up on stodgy cereal and grain-based foods, supplemented by sugary snacks and drinks. Those are the types of foods you should aim to reduce. The main thing you're aiming to do here is to get out of the habit of relying on processed carbohydrates and sugars as a major source of 'nutrition'. After a while it will become second nature, and you'll look back and wonder why on earth you were ever so attached to tasteless, empty foods like pasta and rice.

If all you do is cut out sugar and processed carbohydrates you'll probably find that's enough to make sure your body starts using up your fat reserves while you feel healthier and more energised. But the more closely you follow these guidelines, the better results you will get and the better you will feel.

which foods do you want to wear?

People make all sorts of excuses and try to blame their excess body fat on things that are beyond their control, but usually it's their actions that have caused the fat to be there and it is well within their power to get rid of it. It's not fun to accept responsibility for the excess fat on our bodies, but doing so is an important step on the road to leanness.

In general, people who make mostly healthy food choices look like they make mostly healthy food choices and people who make mostly bad food choices look like they make bad food choices. That's life. So, another question you might want to ask yourself before you eat something is this: 'Do I want to look like someone who eats this type of food?'

If processed carbohydrates and cereals are currently a major part of your diet then I can understand that the idea of cutting them out, even just for 12 weeks, may be causing some concern. But when you take a step back and think about it calmly, it's really only a matter of not adding empty 'filler' to your meals and replacing it with nutritious veggies. You'll be fine.

For example, if you normally have sandwiches for lunch, keep the sandwich filling, but instead of bread have a big bowl of salad. If you buy ready-made mixed salad this will be even quicker to prepare than making a sandwich.

At dinner, you can keep things really interesting by eating a different type of meat or other lean protein source and a different combination of vegetables every night of the week. Cooking meat and steaming or roasting veggies is quick and easy

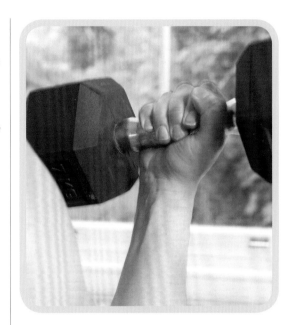

Dreaming about having a great body won't make it a reality. The Fat Burn Revolution programme will.

to prepare and you'll really learn to appreciate the delicious tastes of wholesome vegetables when you stop drenching them in sugar/flour/chemical-filled sauces or gravy.

Eggs make a wonderful breakfast – boiled, poached, scrambled omelette, etc., are all excellent, especially when served with green vegetables

Like the people who have followed the programme before you, you will to learn to make healthier food choices based on the foods you like eating and preparing. If you need more help and advice with this aspect of the programme, visit my website (juliabuckley.co.uk) where you'll find links to places you can get meal ideas and support.

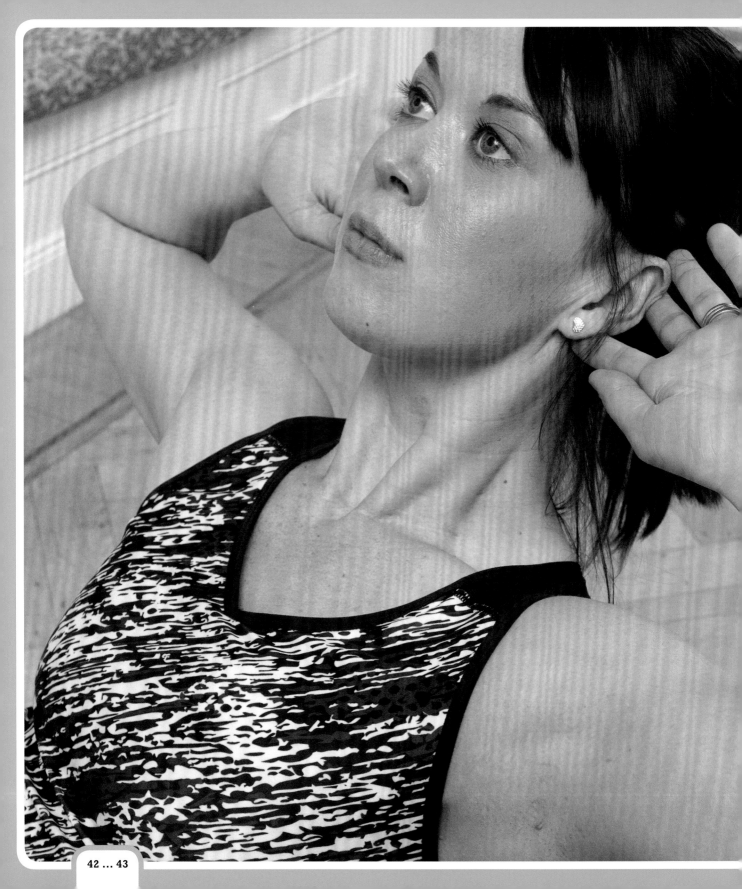

shakes and supplements

I'm not a big fan of taking lots of supplements. It's far better to get your nutrients from food, but they can be handy for helping to fit good nutrition into a busy lifestyle. Personally, I take a daily multivitamin and mineral supplement (which I think of as a sort of insurance policy in case something is missing in my diet that day) an omega-3 (fish oil) supplement (we don't have conclusive proof of all the benefits some people associate with this yet, but the evidence looks pretty good that it is effective in reducing inflammation and aids brain function) and I also use whey protein shakes.

'Hang on there, Julia,' you're probably thinking, 'isn't whey a dairy product?'

Yes, it is... I guess even when you don't have rules you can have exceptions! I'll explain...

Most of the lactose and hormones are removed in the manufacturing process of good whey protein powders, so it's much better than drinking milk. It is still better to get your protein from food if you can, but a whey shake does provide a really useful way to give the body the nutrients it needs in a portable form when food is not a convenient option. Like a lot of people, I use whey shakes to help support my workouts and I'll often throw a shaker cup containing a serving of protein powder into my gym bag. I simply add water to it post-training, down the shake and dash off to my next appointment knowing I've given my body what it needs to recover from the exercise.

A big mistake a lot of people make when exercising for the goal of fat loss is the use of energy

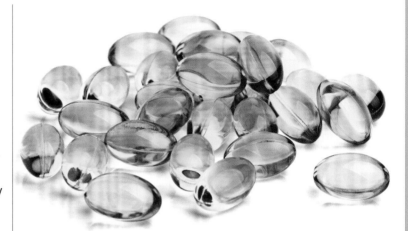

Your food choices will be reflected in the way your body looks, feels and performs.

drinks, gels or bars. Following the dietary guidelines will ensure your body is equipped to tackle the training and tap into its fat stores. Most energy supplements consist mainly of some type of sugar. They can be helpful to long-distance endurance athletes, but you don't need them on this programme and consuming them would be likely to inhibit your fat loss. I do not recommend them for most people taking part in the Fat Burn Revolution.

It's time to leave behind the days of guiltily cramming tasteless, cheap foods into your body. Eating should be a pleasurable activity and knowing that your food is nourishing and helping your body to thrive makes it a much more relaxed and satisfying experience. Bon appetit!

6 gearing up

Now, you understand the principles behind the Fat Burn Revolution, it's time to get ready to put the programme into action.

the gear

The only essential exercise equipment for the training programme is a set of dumbbells and a gym ball (sometimes called a Swiss ball or exercise ball).

dumbbells For the majority of people kitting themselves out for the Fat Burn Revolution, bar-and-plate dumbbell sets are going to be the best option. These come with a pair of bars and a range of circular weight plates with holes in the centre for sliding onto the bars. The plates are then secured on the bars with collars. The two most common types of these are spinlock collars, which screw into place, or clip collars, which expand when you squeeze the levers and snap into place when released. I like the clips because they take less time to get on and off, but the spinlock collars don't take much longer and are a bit more robust, which is worth bearing in mind if you're capable of lifting very heavy weights.

The plates are usually made from either cast iron or concrete encased in plastic or rubber. The cast-iron type are a bit more expensive, but in the long term they're well worth the extra investment. Because metal plates are narrower they take up less space on the bar, leaving room to add more plates on as you get stronger. Another advantage of bar-

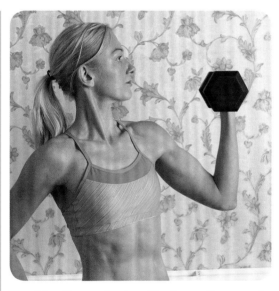

Combine the workouts with close adherence to the eating guidelines and the fat won't stand a chance.

and-plate dumbbells is that they don't take up a lot of space. You can take them apart when you're not using them so they're easy to stow away.

Fixed-weight dumbbells are considerably more expensive for a comprehensive set and require more storage space because you will need several pairs. But they do have the great advantage of not requiring any set up, which reduces time spent making adjustments between exercises. So fixed

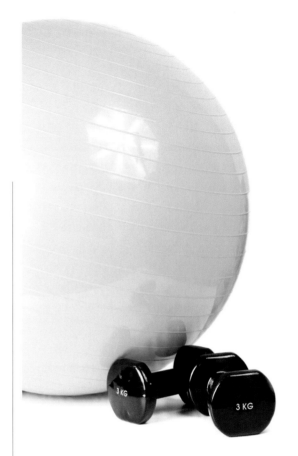

weights are ideal so long as you have access to the right range of weights to challenge yourself. They usually also tend to be a bit more comfortable to hold.

Everyone is different and the weight of the dumbbells you will need to use will depend on the condition of your individual body. Beginners tend to need a set with dumbbell options starting from 3kg pairs up to 10kg pairs to get started. However, you may well find your needs are different. My general recommendation for your starting set-up, if you're buying a bar-and-plate set, is to look for one with a total weight of at least 20kg. If you're buying fixed weight dumbbells don't bother with anything lower than 3kg (single dumbbell weight) and get at least three different pairs. Something like 4kg, 6kg and 9kg pairs will most likely be enough to start you off.

Be aware that you will get stronger, probably quite quickly, and you may well require heavier weights after just a few weeks of doing the Fat Burn Revolution workouts. At the time of writing, suitable bar-and-plate sets are available at around £30–£50. Fixed weight dumbbells at the weights I mentioned would cost around £15–50 per pair (the heavier ones being more expensive, obviously).

So, you will need to invest in weights. But in my opinion a set of dumbbells is the best, most versatile piece of exercise equipment you can buy and there will always be a place for them in your training no matter how far you progress. A half-decent set

> There will be days when you don't feel like doing your workout. Do it anyway. The results will be the same.

should last a lifetime. (I still have a pastel-coloured 3–5kg dumbbell set my grandparents bought me when I was first getting into exercise when I was 17!) Dumbbells are not a gimmicky gadget and, for good reason, have been a staple in every decent gym since the advent of gyms as we know them!

 gym ball Getting yourself a gym ball shouldn't require much investment at all. A 65cm one will be right for most people. At the time of writing these are available for under £10 if you shop around. You'll need this for some of the abdominal and core exercises in Phases II and III, so not until four weeks into the programme if you are following the standard schedule.

other equipment Other useful items are an exercise mat and step or bench. If you don't have these and don't want to invest in them, you can improvise by placing a towel on a well-cushioned floor and lying on that instead of a mat. Instead of a step or bench you can use your stairs at home or, for some exercises, a chair or bench or (sturdy) coffee table will do fine.

Of course, you will also need suitable clothing. It doesn't have to be special fitness gear if you don't have it, just wear something comfortable that you can easily move around in. I recommend

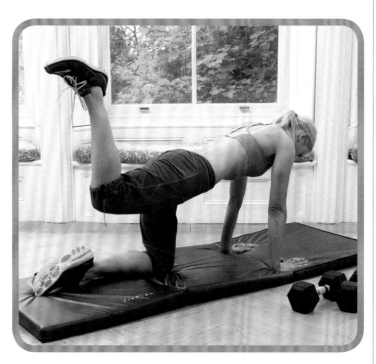

Wear comfortable clothing which allows you to move freely and your skin to breathe.

a good cushioned pair of training shoes for any of the sessions that involve jumping. You can also wear these for sessions that only involve resistance training, but many people (myself included) prefer to wear 'minimalist' thin-soled shoes or to do the sessions with bare feet for maximum stability. For ladies, a well-fitted sports bra is essential – this is one item of specifically designed exercise clothing you should not workout without.

the grub

Once you've got your kit sorted it's time to go grocery shopping. Buy lots of vegetables, and I mean lots! As you know, you'll be cutting right back on cereals and grains (including bread, pasta, rice and pastry), anything containing refined sugar and most dairy products. You will be replacing those with nutrient-filled veggies, fruits and lean proteins (fish, white meat, lean cuts of red meat, eggs, beans and pulses, Quorn, etc.) so stock up!

the gadgets

If you don't have weighing scales and a basic tape measure, it would be a good idea to get hold of some. Body-fat analyser scales can be a useful gadget too. These measure your body-fat percentage as well as weight. Many models also give hydration level and muscle mass estimates. They have their limitations, but they can be a handy way of tracking progress.

Body-fat analyser scales work using what's called bioelectrical impedance analysis. You stand with bare feet on a metal contact area on the scale and the device sends a small, harmless electrical current through your body up from the soles of your feet. Don't worry, it doesn't hurt, although some people report a slight tingling sensation. Because electrical current passes more slowly through fat than muscle the device is able to gauge how much fat is in your body compared to the muscle and thus can estimate what percentage of your body is composed of fat.

However, they are not always reliable and in my experience they seem to work better for some people than others. Readings can be distorted by the amount of water and food in your system, changes in circulation rate (such as following exercise or a stressful experience) and even body temperature. I recommend using them first thing in the morning straight after you get out of bed, that way you'll be keeping conditions as similar as you can each time you step on them. Even though the readings may not be very accurate you can still use them to get a rough idea of your progress.

This brings me to a question I get asked all the time: how often should you step on the scale? I've found that different strategies suit different people, but generally, while people are working towards fat loss I recommend getting on the scales once per day.

Now, I know this may well go against advice you've been given elsewhere and you may be surprised to hear it coming from me, given that I've just explained that I'd prefer you didn't focus too much on weight. So let me explain. There are several reasons I recommend this, firstly, and most importantly, so people can see overall trends in their weight and body-fat levels. As explained, both weight and body-fat readings can fluctuate on a day-to-day basis, so recording them daily allows people to see temporary changes for the blips that they are, rather than getting mistakenly concerned or excited about them. It can also serve as a daily reminder of your goals. Plus it can help you to make the connection between the foods you've been eating

> *It's your body and you are taking control now. That is what the Fat Burn Revolution is all about.*

and the current weight and composition on your body. If you eat too many fattening foods one day and struggle to lose fat for a few days afterwards, you'll have a good idea what might have caused your progress to stall.

Daily weighing may not be for you. It doesn't suit everyone and you are, of course, free to choose whatever weighing protocol you like. In fact, you do not have to use scales at all if you don't want to. Some people prefer just to measure or look at how their clothes fit or take scale readings weekly or even monthly. If something like that is what you think will work best for you, then go with it. But the daily option is there for you if you want it. Just because a lot of popular diet plans/groups/gurus have told you not to, doesn't mean you can't do it now if that's what you want to do. By now you should be fully aware that weight is not necessarily a good gauge of how good you look or how much fat you are carrying and that the numbers will fluctuate daily. You also understand why you're looking for a general trend rather than a daily drop. So, if you are an adult and have no history of eating disorders or obsession with weight then go ahead and step on the scales every morning if you want to. It's your body and you're taking control now. That's what the Fat Burn Revolution is all about.

keeping a journal

I highly recommend you record your experiences, daily diet and workout session details in a journal. If you're a stationery fan you could treat yourself to an attractive notepad that you'll enjoy writing in or if you prefer a keyboard to pen and paper there's digital version available to download at juliabuckley.co.uk.

 Every workout where you lift a heavier weight, complete more repetitions, or do a more advanced version of an exercise than the one before becomes a mini-victory!

Keeping a journal is a very effective, tried-and-tested tool to help you achieve your goals. It forces you to think about what you have and haven't done (or have and haven't eaten). For many people the mere fact that they know they are going to have to write everything they eat down in a journal helps them to eat a better diet. Knowing that they can't just cram foods down their throats and then conveniently forget about it makes them stop and think twice about their food choices. Seeing these details written down somehow makes them seem more 'real' and relevant, which encourages more mindful decision-making.

Secondly, journal keeping can shed light on the cause and effect of your actions. For example, it will show you if there starts to be a pattern where you don't eat properly one day then don't feel like you have the energy to put in a good workout on the next. Or, if you overeat processed foods or drink excessive alcohol one week and then see an increase when you step on the scales and/or measure yourself a few days later, it will be a lot harder to blame it on water retention. It's not so easy to pretend to yourself that you can't understand why the numbers aren't going in the right direction when the evidence is laid bare in front of you.

It's not all 'stick' and no carrot though. The best thing about keeping a Fat Burn Revolution journal is that it's highly motivational and becomes a record of achievement you can be very proud of. As well as logging what you eat, you should also document the details (weights used, rep counts, how you felt, etc.) of each workout you do. One reason for this is to allow you to see the relationship between what you eat and your performance in your workouts. But the fun thing about it is that by recording what you achieve in each of your workouts you will be setting yourself a target to beat in your next session.

If you have a week where the scales do not show any signs of progress, you may still have a victorious workout or two, or vice versa. People often don't notice their fitness and strength improving but seeing the details on paper gives sold proof that their commitment is paying off. On the practical side, it also saves time messing about finding the right weights for each exercise at the start of every session and can also help with meal planning.

Writing things down is a very comforting, cathartic experience for a lot of people too.

Recording your feelings and experiences may help you to stay calm and give you space to remember why you're doing all this. It's important to look back often and appreciate the wonderful changes you're making for yourself and those you care about.

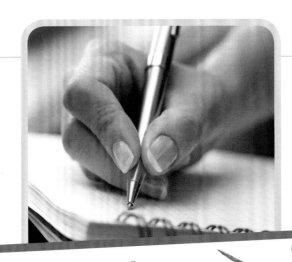

your **workout** journal

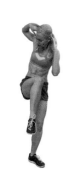

food diary

week	date	food & drink consumed	comments

your **workout** journal

body blaster workout

week	day		date	circuit 1 reps	circuit 2 reps	circuit 3 reps	comments
		push up					
		steam engine					
		star jumps					
		plank					
		burpees					
		step up					

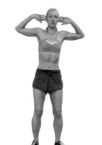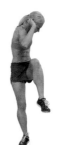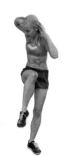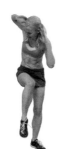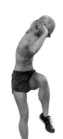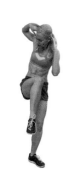

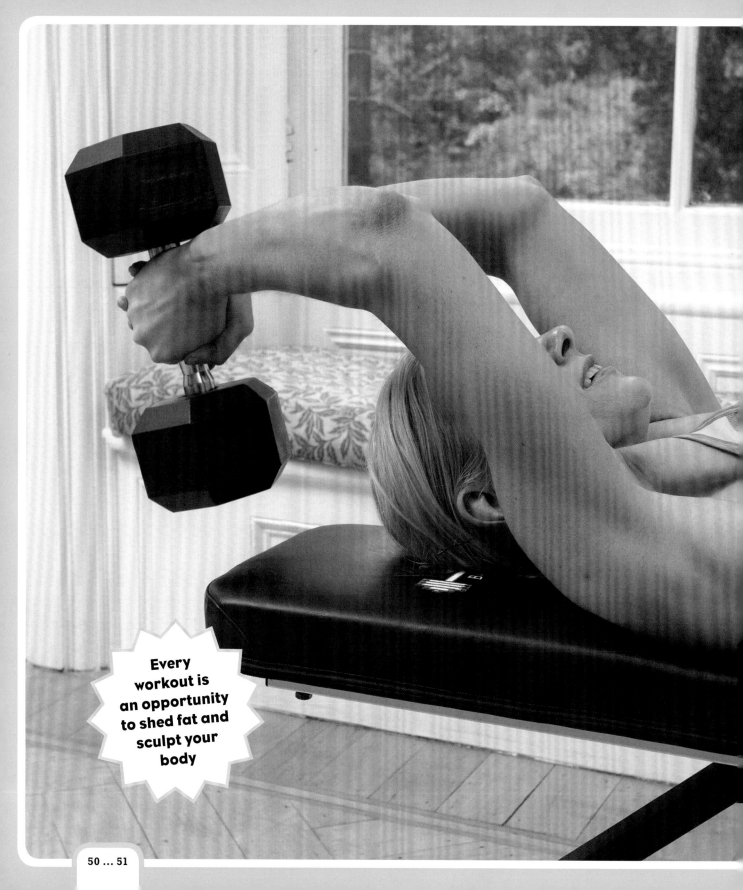

Every workout is an opportunity to shed fat and sculpt your body

the dreaded 'Before' shot

ow it's time to take your Before photo. This is probably not going to be much fun for you, I know. But that's OK, no one likes it, just do it anyway.

Most people hate seeing their Before shot. But I can assure you that they are an incredibly effective aid to fat loss. These images dissolve the fuzz of denial which descends when people tell themselves that their poor diet and lack of exercise doesn't matter. Looking at your Before photo will force you to face the reality of the current condition of your body. But there's no need to be down on yourself if you're shocked or unhappy about what you see. You should smile because now you have leverage that is going to help you make changes. And the benefits of those changes are going to spread far and wide throughout many aspects of your life. This a goodbye photo, remember, you are on the road to the Fat Burn Revolution.

Some of the participants in the pilot programme stored their Before photos on their phones and looked at them whenever the thought of straying off-course entered their heads. Seeing the shots provided a potent reminder of their goals. This worked really well for them. It worked at the beginning of the programme by helping to remind them that they have work to do to get the body they wanted and later in the programme it served as an encouraging reminder of how far they'd come in just a handful of weeks.

You don't have to show the photograph to anyone else if you don't want to. But when you have slimmed down and toned up you may find you want

> Think of your Before photo as part of the process of saying goodbye to the fat you're about to shed.

to share it so other people who are feeling the same way you did at the start can see the changes the Fat Burn Revolution could make to them. When that day comes I'd love to hear from you and will be happy to publish your photos on my website.

But let's not get ahead of ourselves, before that can happen we have work to do!

HERE ARE A FEW TIPS ON TAKING YOUR BEFORE PHOTO:

● WEAR SOMETHING THAT SHOWS A LOT OF FLESH. UNDERWEAR OR SWIMSUITS ARE IDEAL

● STAND SOMEWHERE WITH A PLAIN, UNCLUTTERED BACKDROP

● TAKE LOTS OF SHOTS IN DIFFERENT POSES. FACING FRONT, BACK, TO THE SIDES, HANDS UP, HANDS AT SIDES, HANDS ON HIPS, AND ANY MORE YOU CAN THINK OF

● STAND IN A NATURAL POSTURE. NO SUCKING THE BELLY IN OR PUSHING THE CHEST OUT

● DON'T WORRY ABOUT TRYING TO MAKE THE PICTURE FLATTERING, THIS IS PART OF YOUR FAT BURN REVOLUTION AND IT NEEDS TO BE REAL. YOU MAY NOT ENJOY DOING THIS NOW, BUT YOU'RE GOING TO BE VERY GLAD YOU HAVE THESE PHOTOS IN JUST A FEW MONTHS

7 the nitty gritty

Now your mind is in the right place to start the Fat Burn Revolution, and now that you've gathered all the kit you need, it's time to get down to the nitty gritty. In this chapter I'll tell you what to expect from the workouts and why they form part of the optimal recipe for fat-burning fitness.

If you have exercised with weights before or done any boot camp or military-style training, some of the moves will probably be familiar to you. But even if you haven't done any of the exercises before there's nothing to worry about, all will be explained and illustrated with photos.

Metabolic Resistance Workouts

Throughout the three four-week phases of the Fat Burn Revolution, you'll be doing two to three Metabolic Workout sessions per week. In these you'll use either dumbbells or your own bodyweight to create resistance to challenge the muscles of your body. These sessions are not about moving fast or performing lots of repetitive movements: you'll be lifting weights which are quite heavy (whatever that means for you) in a slow and controlled manner. The

exercises are grouped into two or three moves per section and you'll complete most of the exercises 10 to 15 times before moving on to the next. This would be described in exercise jargon as 10–15 repetitions, or reps, per set. Once you've finished all of your repetitions of an exercise you'll move onto the next exercise set and you won't take a break until you've completed all the sets of exercises in that section. When each section is complete you'll get a minute of rest to recover before moving on to either repeat the section or start the next one.

Furnace Workouts

In the Furnace Workouts you'll be doing short bursts of hard, fast, cardiovascular training. This will get your heart pumping quickly, your blood circulating, and your lungs working hard to supply your body with the oxygen it needs to perform well. Often called high-intensity interval training (HIIT) this type of exercising has been shown to produce outstanding results both in fat loss and improving fitness, sports performance and health. You're free to choose the type of exercise you'd like to do in

When you're in great physical condition it feels like nothing in life can hold you down.

As you strip back the fat, lean muscle will be revealed, giving you a sexy, sculpted shape.

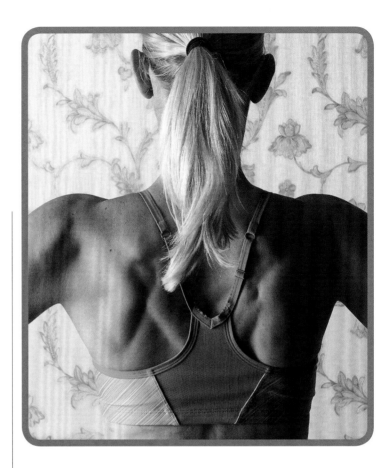

these sessions. It just needs to be something that doesn't require a lot of coordination, but provides a challenging workout for you if performed at close to your maximum speed for short periods of time. My favoured method is to do these on a stationary exercise bike, as I believe this provides the optimal balance of safety and toughness, but a lot people prefer running, cycling, swimming or fast-moving bodyweight exercises, e.g. burpees or mountain climbers (described in Chapter 8).

If you're not performing your intervals on a machine or in front of a clock, it could be useful to get an interval bleeper. Some sports watches have this function or there are several free interval timer apps available that you can download onto your smartphone. You'll find links to some of them at juliabuckley.co.uk.

Total Body Blast

The Total Body Blast is a full body workout. It requires no equipment, which makes it very handy for when you're away from home without access to a gym. You'll do this workout once per week in Phase I of the Fat Burn Revolution and you'll also have option of using it in Phase II. There are only six exercises to learn for this workout and there is no target rep count. You will simply perform each exercise for 30 seconds and record the number of repetitions you do in your journal (with a view to increasing that number each week). You'll go through

all six exercises, take a break and repeat for a total of three circuits. Sound easy? It's not. But it is well worth it – these sessions burn serious flab!

Metabolic Blaster

In Phase II we'll shake things up a bit by combining one of your resistance training sessions with some high-intensity plyometric moves. Plyometric training uses quick, explosive movements, so you'll be building power and agility as well as strength. This workout will 'shock' your body with a brand-new way of training and has tremendous fat-burning potential if you give it your all. If you have joint problems or a lot of excess weight the full plyometric versions of the moves might not be for you, but that's fine, you have the option of doing them as non-plyo cardio exercises.

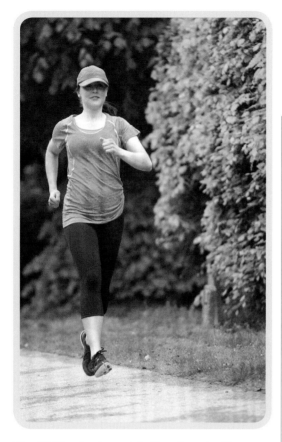

The 20-30 minute metabolism boost will stoke your metabolism and help optimise fat burning throughout the day.

Plyo Blaze

By Phase III you'll be ready to take things up another gear. One place you definitely notice this is the Plyo Blaze workout. You were introduced to plyometric training in Phase II and now you will take on a full session of fast-paced explosive exercise. This workout will really help torch the gristle – it's like throwing petrol on your metabolic fire! You will find it very challenging at first, but one of the best things about this type of exercise is that people tend to adapt quite quickly to it, so although it will never be an easy session, you find it becomes much more manageable as you progress. Again, you can substitute low-impact moves if there's any reason why plyometric exercise might not be wise for you.

Belly Shred

In the final phase of the programme you will do the Belly Shred workout three times per week. I suggest you add it to the end of your Metabolic Workout sessions. This workout only takes about 20 minutes to do and targets your core and stomach muscles to ensure that when you strip back those final layers of flab, a flat, defined abdominal area will be revealed.

20–30 minute metabolism booster

For optimal results you should also do 20–30 minutes of sustained low-intensity exercise at least six hours either before or after your workout session of the day. This can anything that gets you moving – walking, jogging, swimming, dancing, Pilates, gardening, housework, shopping, etc., are all fine.

People tend to compensate for workouts by being less generally active during the rest of the day. Often they don't even realise it, they just don't get up and move around as much. This will help to make sure you don't fall into that trap. As the name suggests, your metabolism will get an extra boost, which will ensure you keep fat burning going all day long. Plus you'll be adding into your daily routine some type of relaxing activity that you already enjoy. If you have an active job where you're already moving around a lot during your working day anyway then you don't have to do this, in fact, it would be better for you rest up ready for your next workout session.

max-ing the burn

I want you to get the best possible results in return for the time and effort you put into the Fat Burn revolution. From start to finish you should aim to consistently push yourself beyond your previous limits whenever you can to get the full benefit of the programme.

In many of the sessions you're going to be reaching the point of what is called failure. In the Fat Burn Revolution this is a positive thing, as in many other of life's endeavours, true success comes only after you've experienced failure!

I'm certainly not talking about performing the moves incorrectly here, but rather about exercising with good form to the point where you cannot continue while maintaining the proper technique and posture. Most of the exercises in the metabolic workouts engage many muscles across the body (which is another reason why they are so effective for fat loss) as other muscles come into play to support the movements of the main target muscles for each exercise. As failure approaches you may experience a shakiness throughout your whole body, often mainly in the muscles in your midsection, or core. Soon after that you'll struggle to maintain good posture and/or movement patterns, which means it's time to stop and either rest or move onto the next exercise. Other times failure may be specific to the exercise's main target areas, which will start to ache and wobble as those muscles approach their maximum work threshold.

To reach this point you'll need to use a weight that is relatively heavy for you. If the stated number of repetitions for an exercise is, for example, 10, you should be at the point where you're really struggling by the time you reach your tenth rep, if not before. It's better to only do eight or nine and reach failure at that point than to comfortably bang out 10 with a weight that doesn't present a challenge.

You won't get it right every time, but try to use

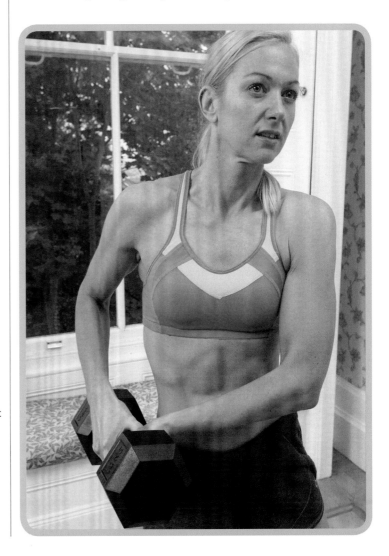

weights that will take you to around the point of failure at the stated number of reps — and no more.

The human body responds really well to this type of training and if it is new to you, you can expect to make a lot of improvements in your fitness and strength over the course of the programme.

Once you can complete the stated number of reps for any of the exercises it is time to increase the weight or perform a more advanced version of the move. This is a much better approach than adding on extra reps. Occasionally you might misjudge the weight you need and find you don't get much of a challenge from the stated number of reps. If that happens you could add in a few extra, but this should not be a regular occurrence. Record what happened in your journal and ensure you pick the right weight next time so you can get maximum benefits from your session.

As mentioned in Chapter 3, the word 'metabolic' is used a lot in describing the programme because of the 'afterburn' effect you benefit from with this type of training – that is, your body continues to use up more fat long after the session. This programme

> If you haven't exercised this way before it may take a while for you to get used to it and to learn not to be afraid to push to the point of failure. But you will find that by doing this your strength, fitness and body shape will improve faster than you have ever experienced before.

Recording your session in your journal is key to making the most of every workout and getting optimal results from the programme.

is not about working in your 'comfort zone'. You may well have witnessed all those people who spend hours in the gym doing tons of repetitions with weights or long sessions on cardio machines yet still can't shake off body fat. Maybe you know that feeling of frustration very well already. This programme is different: we go harder, not longer – because that's what makes fat burning and fitness gains happen.

planning your Revolution

Now you know what you're in for, let's talk about putting the Fat Burn Revolution exercise plan into action. Forward planning is one of the most powerful weapons you have in your war on excess body fat, so use it well. I recommend scheduling all of your training sessions for the week ahead every Sunday. You can use your journal for this, but I recommend you also enter them in your main/professional daily diary or planner. You have to get into the mindset of thinking of your workouts as important appointments that are set in stone. Unless something really important comes up, you should not miss or move them. For example, a friend coming over to visit or an invitation to post-work drinks should not be enough to make you waiver, but taking someone to hospital is excusable! Keep reminding yourself that you are going for maximum results during the programme. In less than three months' time (if you're following the standard 12-week schedule), when you've finished the programme, you can start being a bit more flexible if that feels right for you. But at least until then, while you establish and embed your new routine, you need to give exercise a very high place in your list of priorities.

The Fat Burn Revolution is suitable for people with a wide range of fitness levels, but whatever level you're at you should start from Phase I of the programme and work through to Phase III. Give yourself at least four weeks on each phase before moving on to the next. Even if you already do some of the exercises that are included in Phase I regularly, if you follow the programme properly, the workouts will not be easy because you will be using weights that take you to the point of failure in the Metabolic sessions and working at your maximum threshold in the Body Blaster circuit and the Furnace interval sessions. Wherever your limits are, you will be pushing them.

You can schedule the sessions to suit your lifestyle, but I will suggest which workouts to do on which days at the start of the next three chapters. I recommend at least one rest day per week or at

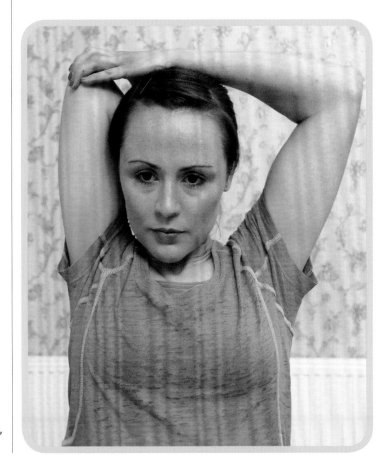

least two if you're new to regular exercise. Feel free to take additional rest days if you feel unwell or find the schedule is leaving you over-tired. Do not perform the same workout on two consecutive days as this will inhibit recovery. (If you are using the correct weights this would be a highly uncomfortable thing to do anyway!)

Rest days should not be completely sedentary. Keep those metabolic fires burning by including light activity in your day, aiming to complete at least half an hour of continuous, low-intensity exercise. Again, this can be anything that gets you moving (e.g. walking, jogging, swimming, dancing, gentle yoga or Pilates, gardening, housework, shopping, etc.).

what if I miss a planned session?

You missed a workout? Shame on you, you've undone all your good work, so you might as well just forget the whole thing and go eat a big sugar pie – just kidding!

Of course, the opposite is true. One missed session won't really set you back and is nothing to worry about all, so long as it doesn't become a habit. If you catch yourself thinking of using a missed session as an excuse to miss further workouts, that's when you need to sit down and have a rational word with yourself!

The thing to do is get back to the programme the following day, ideally starting with the session you missed. But if this makes rescheduling difficult you could just leave out that session entirely and resolve to push extra hard in that workout next week. You can probably get away with doing that once per four-week phase, but try not to exceed that or it may affect your progress, especially in the case of the Metabolic, Belly Shred and Plyo Blaze workouts.

Sometimes exercises which you find challenging might make you feel mal-coordinated or weak – this will make it all the more satisfying when you find yourself getting stronger.

You only get the chance to do each workout four times at most: miss one of those sessions and you've missed 25% of that aspect of the training. I don't recommend trying to catch up by doing more than one session per day, it is much better to put all of your energy into a single workout.

what if I miss several sessions?

If you veer off course for several days or more it's even more important not to get down on yourself. It may be tough to get back on course if you feel you've lost momentum, but do it anyway and you'll soon be very glad you did. It may mean it will take a little longer to get to where you want to be, but just think of it as a bend in the road. If you've missed a week or less, I recommend picking up the programme where you left off. If you've missed a longer period you may need to restart earlier in the programme so you can remind yourself of the moves and regain lost fitness, but you should find it returns very quickly.

On days when you do miss exercise, it is especially important to keep your diet clean. This will help avoid your results going in the wrong direction and make it easier to get back on track with the workouts. It will also help you stay in the correct mindset.

If you have any more questions you'd like to get answered before starting The Fat Burn Revolution visit my website juliabuckley.co.uk and I'll point you in the right direction.

Got all the info you need? Then get ready to change your body and change your life.

work your weaknesses

WE ALL HAVE SOME EXERCISES THAT WE LIKE TO DO MORE THAN OTHERS AND USUALLY THE EXERCISES WE LIKE TO DO ARE THE ONES WE ARE GOOD AT. WHAT I MEAN BY THAT IS THE EXERCISES WHERE WE DON'T STRUGGLE TO MAINTAIN GOOD FORM AND/OR PERFORM ADVANCED VERSIONS AND/OR USE A DECENT AMOUNT OF WEIGHT. EXERCISES THAT HIT OUR WEAK SPOTS OR CAUSE US TO WOBBLE AND WAIVER CAN MAKE US FEEL WEAK AND MALCOORDINATED, WHICH MOST OF US DON'T ENJOY AT ALL.

IT'S TOTALLY UNDERSTANDABLE: WE ALL FEEL BETTER DOING SOMETHING WE CAN DO WELL THAN DOING SOMETHING WE CAN'T. BUT I DON'T THINK I NEED TO TELL YOU WHICH OF THOSE LEADS TO THE BEST IMPROVEMENTS IN YOUR BODY!

TRY TO HAVE FUN WITH IT. MOST PEOPLE HAVE TO GO THROUGH BEING BAD AT AN EXERCISE BEFORE THEY CAN BECOME GOOD AT IT. TAKE YOUR TIME AND REALLY FOCUS WHEN PERFORMING THE EXERCISES YOU'RE WEAKER AT AND, ALTHOUGH THEY MIGHT NEVER BECOME YOUR FAVOURITE MOVES, YOU WILL GRADUALLY GAIN MASTERY OVER THEM AND YOU'LL LEARN TO ENJOY THEM MORE. BEING DRIVEN TO IMPROVE ON YOUR WEAKNESSES IS A HIGHLY BENEFICIAL ATTITUDE TO HAVE, BOTH IN YOUR FITNESS TRAINING AND IN LIFE – AND THIS IS THE PERFECT OPPORTUNITY TO START GETTING INTO THE HABIT.

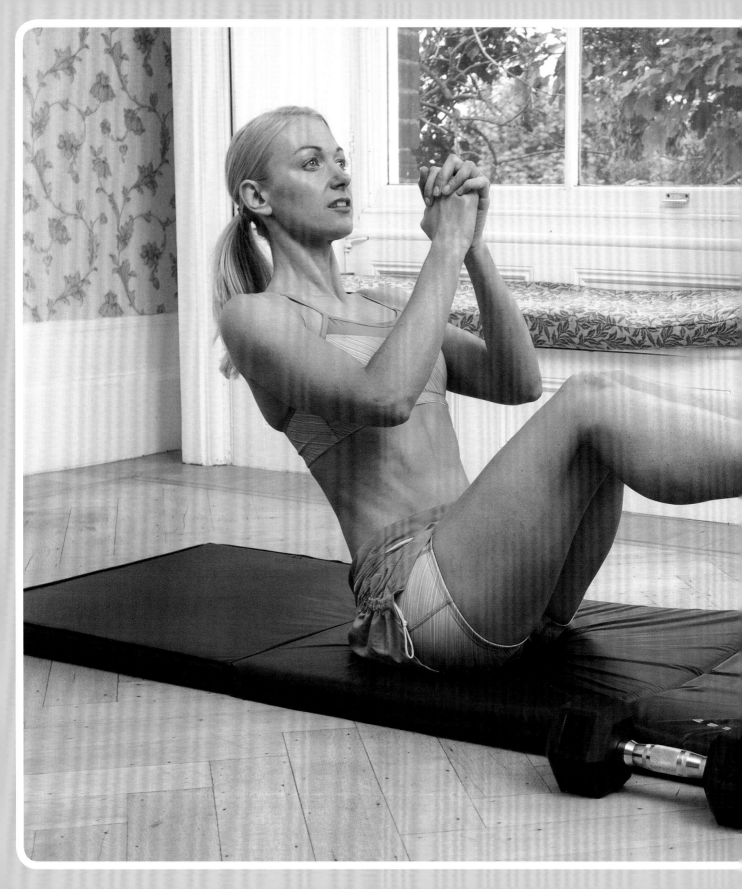

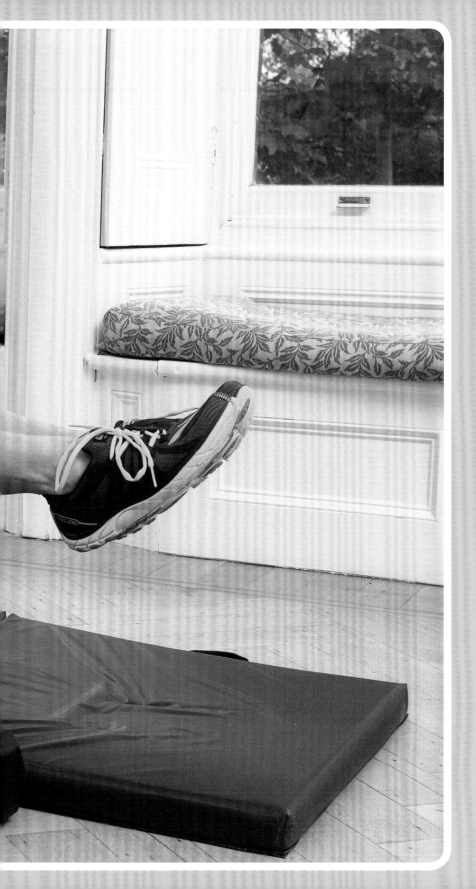

the time for **action** has arrived

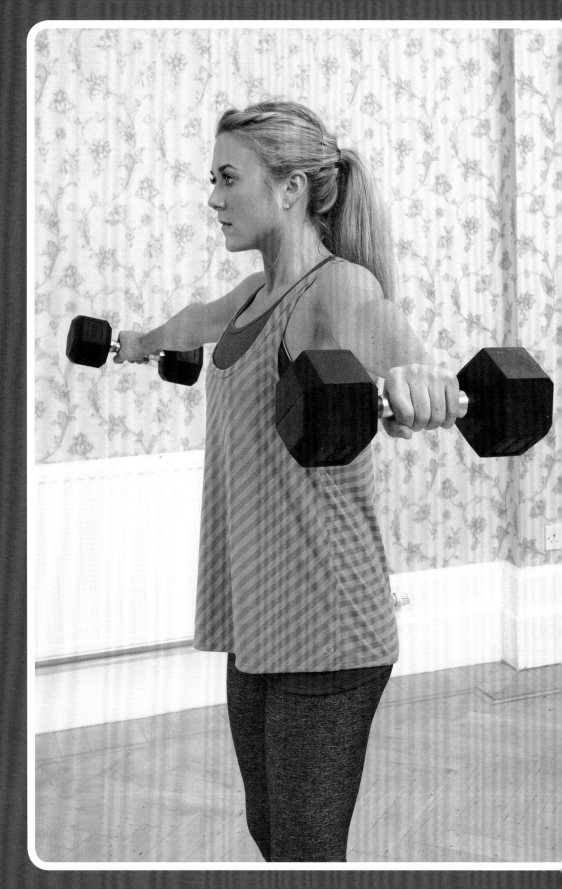

WE'RE ALMOST READY TO GO, BUT BEFORE YOU DIVE IN, PLEASE TAKE NOTE OF THESE SAFETY POINTS:

● Always read through all the materials for each phase of the programme before trying the workouts for the first time.

● If in doubt, don't. If you have any injuries or illnesses which could be exacerbated by performing any of the exercises, or if you're pregnant or on medication, seek advice from a medical professional before starting.

● Any time you're unsure about any aspect of the workouts refer back to the book and if you still don't find the answer you can contact me via my website, juliabuckley.co.uk.

● Don't miss out the tips section at the bottom of each exercise description, these contain important safety notes as well as advice for getting maximum benefits from the moves.

● Exercise in a safe space. This programme is designed to be followed at home, but you must ensure the area where you train is free of objects that you could trip on or bang into and that the floor is not slippery.

● Keep your equipment clean and well maintained and check it over before every session. Collars on dumbbells can become loose quite quickly, so always re-tighten them before starting a workout.

● Many of the exercises will be physically challenging, but they should never be painful. If you feel pain, stop immediately and seek advice from a medical professional.

● The same goes if you feel ill or faint during your workout. Stop right away and see your doctor.

● Keep a glass of water handy and take regular sips to ensure you stay hydrated during the workouts.

● Form is king. When you reach a point in any exercise where you can't continue with good posture and technique then it's time to stop.

a few key terms

repetitions or reps: The number of times you do each individual exercise is counted in repetitions, or reps for short. One repetition is complete when you have performed all stages of the movement and are ready to repeat it or finish your set.

sets: The duration or total number of repetitions in any single exercise is called a set. Most of the exercises in the Fat Burn Revolution are organised into one to three sets, each comprised of 10 repetitions.

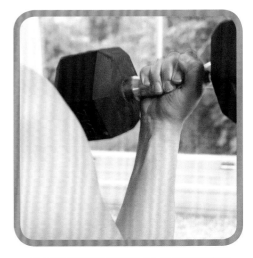

core muscles: Many of the exercises focus on the muscles in the midsection of the body. I use the term 'core' when describing these. The core comprises the muscles in and around the belly (transversus abdominis, internal and external obliques, rectus abdominis) the lower back (multifidus, erector spinae and latissimus dorsi) and often the pelvic floor muscles. Many of these exercises will also activate the gluteal muscles in the bum and trapezius in the upper back.

tightening the core: Keeping your core muscles 'tight' is important in many of the exercises. What I mean by this is that you should contract the muscles of the core without releasing while doing the exercise. Performing the plank exercise will give you an introduction to how this should feel if it is new to you.

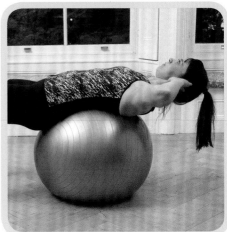

warming up and cooling down

You should always take a few minutes to warm up to get the body ready for exercise. This will help you to perform at your best, reduce the risk of injury and get you in the right frame of mind for the session. For the first part of the warm up I recommend 5–10 minutes of cardiovascular exercise (or longer if you feel you need it). I leave this open for people to choose whatever activity they like. So, for example you could do jogging in place, fast-marching up and down stairs, aerobics-style moves, or working at a moderate pace on an exercise bike, treadmill, rower or other cardio machine. Anything that gets your heart pumping and speeds up your breathing is good, but try to avoid exercises that involve jumping until your joints have had time to warm up and become lubricated.

Once that's done you should perform the dynamic (moving) stretches described in the next section. For the workouts that focus on the upper body you only need to do the upper body dynamic stretches and for the lower-body workouts you only need to do the lower-body dynamic stretches. For the full body sessions (Total Body Blast, Metabolic Blaster and Plyo Blaze) you should do all of them.

The same applies to the post-workout static stretches. The time to perform static (still) stretches is after exercise while your body is cooling down. These will help keep your muscles in good condition and may reduce post-exercise soreness. Pay particular attention to any muscles that feel tight or where you felt a burning sensation in during the workout.

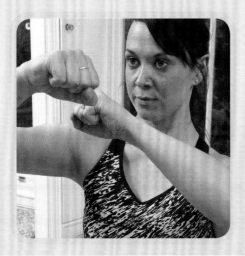
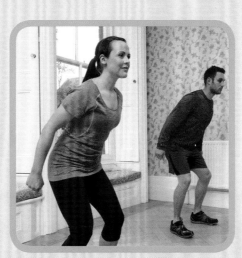

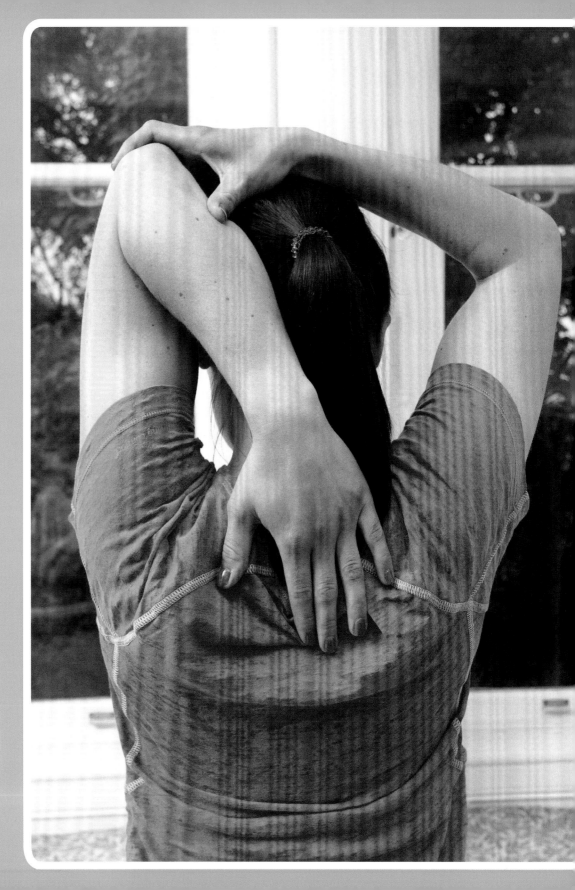

pre-workout dynamic stretches for the upper body

arm circles

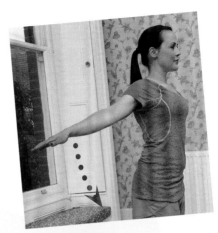

target area
chest, upper back, shoulders

Arm circles are a simple upper-body dynamic stretching exercise to prepare your chest, upper back, and shoulder muscles to work out.

1 Stand tall, keeping your core tight and head facing forward. Relax your arms, shoulders and chest. You may want to loosely waggle and swing your arms to release any tension you could be holding in those areas.

2 Maintaining a straight posture, swing one arm forwards in a circular motion. Stay relaxed, but control the movement, only bringing the arms up to a point that is comfortable for your shoulders. Continue for around 10–12 repetitions or until the area feels warm and loose. Repeat with the other arm.

3 Repeat, but reverse the movement swinging each arm in a backward circle.

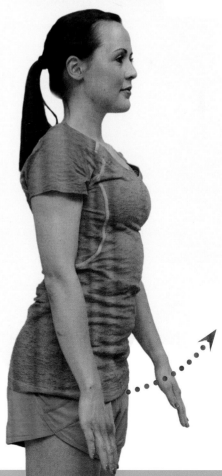

TIPS

Breathe deeply and stay relaxed in the shoulders

Make the movements slow and controlled

Keep your back straight and your head still, only your arms should be moving

This should never be painful, only go to a level where you feel a gentle stretch

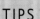

huggers

Huggers are great for preparing the chest, upper back, and shoulder muscles for exercise. They are easy and fun to perform and will help you to feel energised and ready to start your workout.

1 Stand with your feet hip-width apart and raise your arms to chest level. Bend your elbows a little and squeeze your arms together until your fingers are touching as if you were hugging a thick tree trunk! Feel the stretch across your upper back.

2 Bring your arms apart again and now press them back to transfer the stretch into your chest. Palms should be facing upwards at shoulder height. Press your chest forward and shoulders back.

3 Slowly repeat the movement, pausing and holding the stretch for a couple of seconds at either extreme. Continue for at least 10 repetitions.

TIPS

Breathe in as you open your arms, exhale as you hug

Only open your arms to a point where you feel a comfortable stretch

Avoid throwing your arms open or using momentum when swinging them back around you

Remember, the movement should be slow and controlled

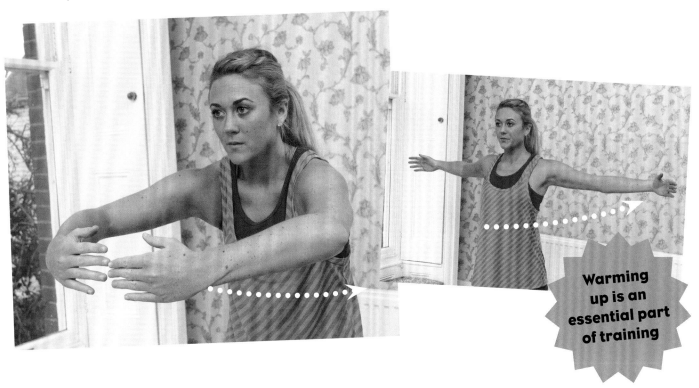

Warming up is an essential part of training

shoulder rolls

A favourite with swimmers, shoulder rolls loosen and warm up the shoulder and upper back muscles. As well as being a good warm up move, this stretch can be helpful any time your neck and shoulders feel tight.

1 Stand tall, feet hip-width apart and let your arms dangle loosely at your sides. Relax the shoulders and neck.

2 With your back straight, head facing forward, lift both of your shoulders up towards your ears and then slowly lower them in a forward circular motion. Repeat this movement 10 times.

3 Return to the starting position and then perform the same movement, but this time rotating the shoulders backwards. Perform this movement 10 times.

target area
shoulders & upper back

TIPS

Breathe deeply and keep the shoulders and neck relaxed

All movements should be done in a slow and controlled manner

Keep your back straight and your chin up, the head and neck should not move

Really concentrate on feeling the stretch throughout each slow rotation

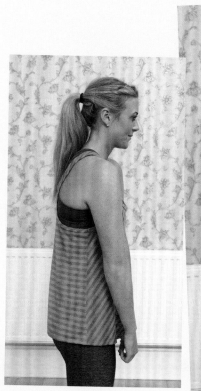
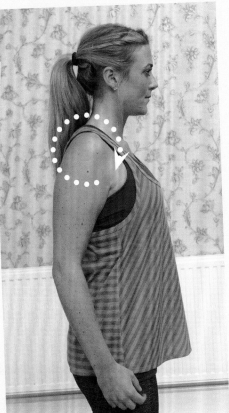
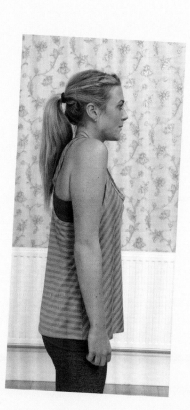

neck rotation

The neck is often forgotten when it comes to warming up the body, which is unfortunate because even though it isn't actively involved in exercise, a lot of tension can build up in this area making the neck prone to strains and stiffness. You can use this exercise anywhere, anytime you feel your tightness in your shoulders and neck.

1 Stand with your feet hip-width apart and let your arms hang loosely at your sides, shoulders relaxed. Tilt your head to the left, pressing the chin towards your shoulder until you feel a comfortable stretch in the neck (and no further).

2 From there, gently lower your chin to your chest and rotate your head upwards tilting over the right shoulder.

3 Repeat in the opposite direction, alternating for 10 repetitions.

TIPS

Breathe deeply and keep your body relaxed

Do not allow the shoulders to hunch up

This stretch should be very gentle, so don't force it and keep the motion very slow

Do not tilt the head backwards

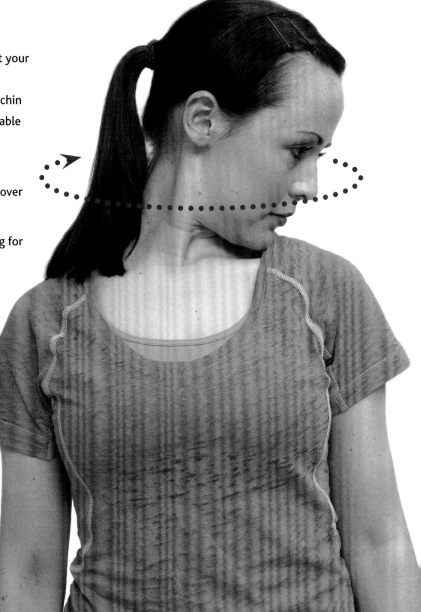

Approach your workouts with a positive attitude. Remember, you don't HAVE to exercise you GET to exercise.

pre-workout dynamic stretches for the lower body

side leg swings

Leg swings are a simple dynamic stretch to prepare the muscles of the thighs and lower back for exercise. Being quite a gentle stretch, this is a nice one to do as your first lower-body stretch of the session.

1 You'll probably need to hold onto something for balance for this exercise, so stand behind something sturdy and stable, or in front of a wall, holding on with one hand. Stand tall, with a straight back, core muscles engaged. Shift your balance onto one leg and raise the other leg out in front of you, a few inches off the floor.

2 Slowly and gently swing the lifted leg out the side, only rising to a comfortable level where you will feel a light stretch in your inner thigh.

3 From there swing your leg back in front of you and across the other leg, again reaching out to the side up to a level where you feel a comfortable stretch. Repeat the movement at least 10 times and then change legs.

target area
thighs

TIPS

Your upper body should be upright at all times and your head facing forward

Use very controlled deliberate movements, do not use momentum to swing the leg like a pendulum

Keep your foot flexed as you swing the leg and do not bend the knee

Never stretch beyond a comfortable level, this should not be painful

Enjoy and appreciate being able to move your body

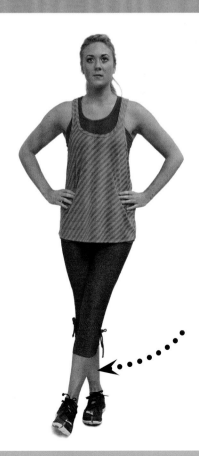

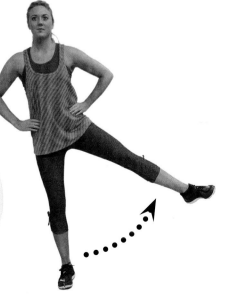

front and back leg swings

This dynamic stretch will wake up and loosen the muscles of the buttocks and thighs in preparation for lower-body exercises.

1 Stand with feet together alongside a table, wall or any stable object that you can hold onto to keep you steady as you balance on one leg. Your head should be facing forward and your back straight – maintain this posture throughout the exercise.

2 Slowly swing the free leg forward and up in front of you to a level where you feel a light stretch in the muscles at the back of the thighs.

3 Now gently swing your leg back out behind you, again only to the point of a comfortable stretch – this time you should feel it in the front of your thighs. Repeat this movement at least 10 times before changing legs.

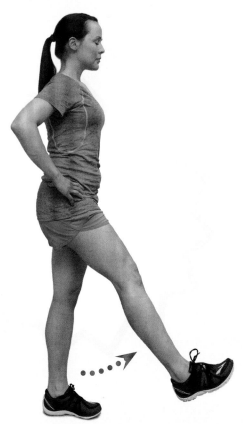
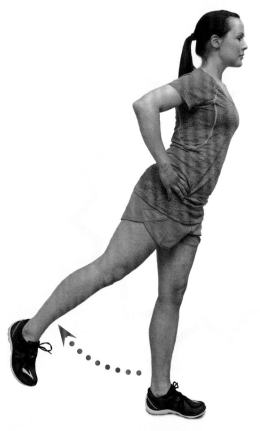

hip circles

target area
hips & lower back

Hip circles are a classic dynamic stretch to help loosen the muscles around the hips and lower back. If you feel a bit stiff or the movement is jerky at first don't worry, that's quite common, you'll be winding like a belly dancer after practicing for a few weeks!

1 Stand with your feet shoulder-width apart and your hands on your hips, keep your head up, look straight out in front of you.

2 Begin circling your hips in a clockwise direction, shifting your weight onto your right foot as you move them to the right and then onto the left foot as you rotate over to the left.

3 Perform 10–12 repetitions in this direction and then repeat in an anti-clockwise direction.

TIPS

Feel free to perform more than 12 repetitions if you feel you need to, many people get quite tight in the hips and it's a great idea to loosen up this area before exercising

Move very slowly, think about exaggerating each phase of the movement to really feel the stretch

Avoid stretching beyond a comfortable level, this should never be painful

Keep your back straight, core tight and head up while you perform this stretch

Look after your body, it's the only one you have!

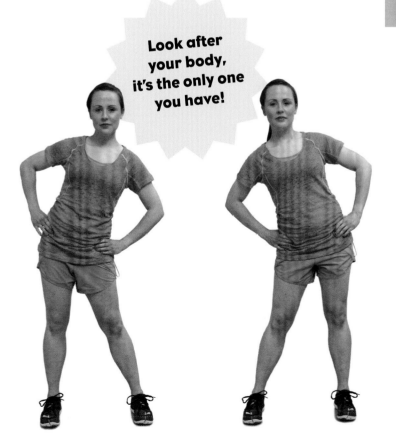
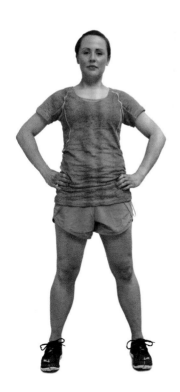

calf step back

This dynamic stretch targets the calf muscles in the lower leg, which often get tight with regular training and can be prone to strains and tears if not properly looked after and warmed up before you start exercising.

1 Start with the feet together, hands on hips. Step backwards with one leg, bending the front knee and keeping the back leg straight.

2 Keeping your back straight and your core tight, activate the stretch by pressing the back heel down to the floor before returning to the start position. Repeat 10 times and switch legs.

3 Now take a short step back and bend both knees. Allow your hips to drop toward the floor, but keep the pelvis tucked forward as you 'sit into' the stretch, feeling it lower down your calf. Repeat 10 times and switch legs.

Warming up preps the body and mind for action

TIPS

The length of your stride will depend on how tight your calf muscle is. Try stepping half a metre behind you at first and extend further back until you feel a stretch

In Step 3 you only need to take a short step backwards, try about 30cm to start with

Feet and knees should stay pointed forward at all times

Keep your knees in-line with ankles, don't let them flare inwards or outwards.

lunge walks

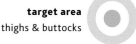

This dynamic stretch may look like a silly walk, but it's actually one of the smartest moves you can do to prepare your whole lower body for exercise.

1 Stand tall and straight with your feet together, firmly planted on the floor. Place your hands on your hips.

2 Take a big step forward and slowly lower your upper body between your legs, bending both of your knees, keeping your hips facing forward, pelvis tucked under. Your aim is to get a 90-degree angle in both legs at the bottom of the stretch, but you should only drop to a point where you feel the stretch, not pain, so you may not be able to get that low at first.

3 Press the feet into the floor as you raise your body back up. Step the back leg in to meet the front leg and then step forward again with the opposite leg and repeat Step 2. Or, if you don't have much space, return the front leg to the starting position and repeat with the opposite leg. Step forwards with alternate legs for a total of 20 lunge strides.

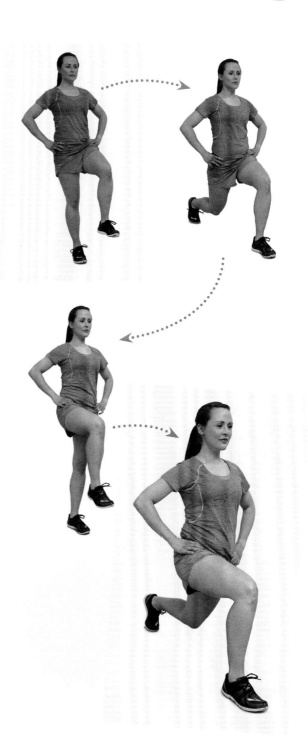

TIPS

Both feet should be pointed forward at all times

Avoid stretching beyond a comfortable level, you should never feel pain

Do not allow your knees to flare inwards or outwards, keep them in-line with your feet and ankles throughout the exercise

Your front foot should be flat on the floor as you lower down, balancing on the ball of your back foot

post-workout static stretches for the upper body

bicep stretch

target area
upper arm

The bicep muscles in the front of the upper arm can get sore and stiff after a hard workout. This move helps decrease the muscle soreness and keep your arms loose and flexible.

1 Stand straight with your feet hip-width apart. Lift your arms out from your sides so they're at about a 45-degree angle to your torso.

2 Keeping your arms straight, palms open, extend and reach diagonally downwards until you feel a good stretch in the upper arms. Hold for 30 seconds.

3 Turn your wrists so your palms are facing behind you, thumbs pointing to the floor and again reach until you feel the stretch. Hold for 30 seconds.

TIPS

Do not bend the arms at the elbows or wrists

Do not allow the shoulders to hunch up

Keep the back straight – if you feel it start to arch, think about tucking your pelvis under

Breathe deeply as you hold the stretch

Getting started can be the hardest part of working out, some days you just have to turn your mind off and begin.

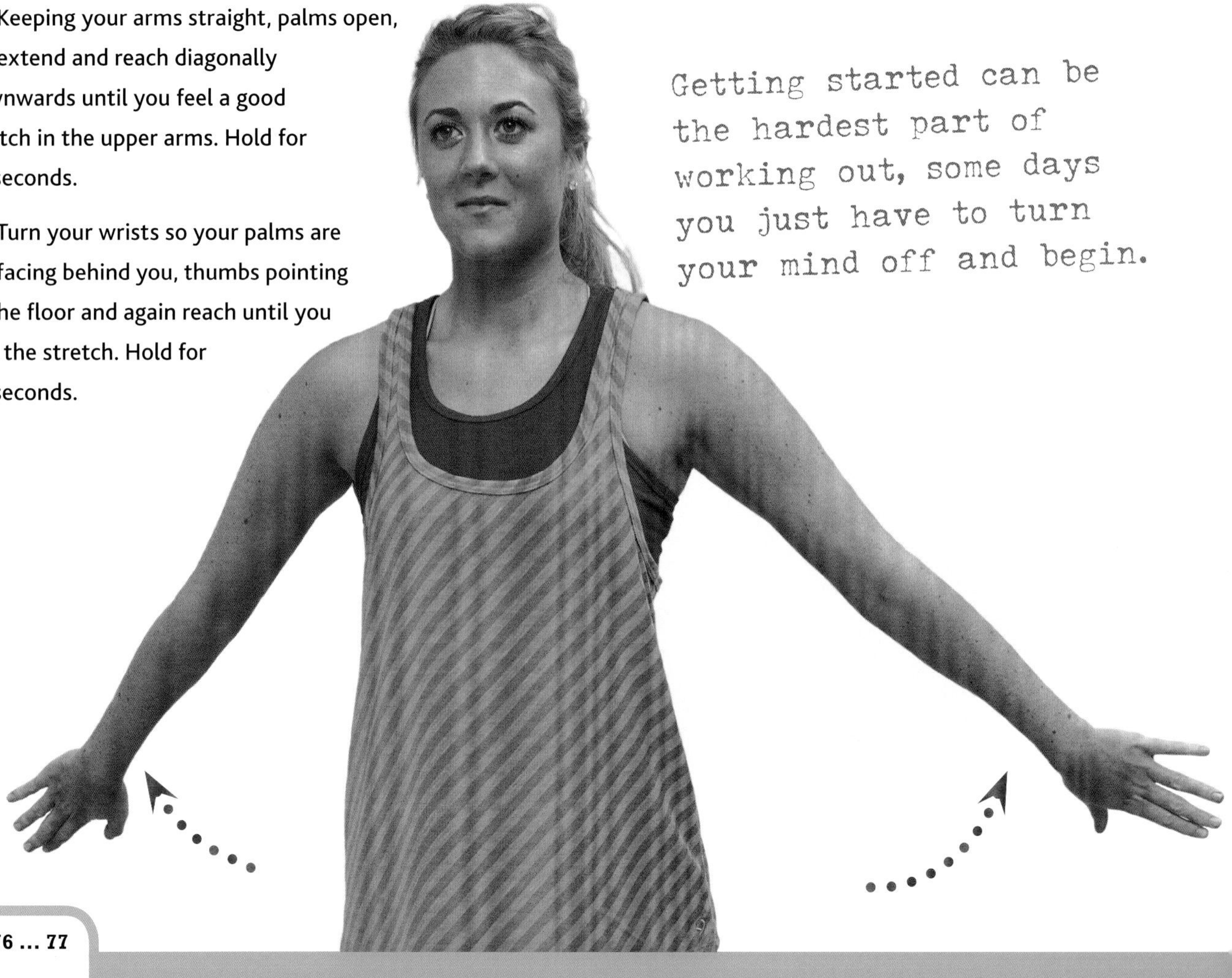

overhead tricep stretch

Like the biceps on the front of the upper arm, the triceps on the back of the arm can be prone to soreness after a tough workout, this move will help minimise that as well as keeping the muscle flexible and less prone to injury, it also gives your upper back a stretch.

1 Stand tall with your feet hip-width apart and your arms at your sides. Raise one arm, bend the elbow and place the palm of your hand behind your neck or, if you can reach, on your upper back between your shoulder blades.

2 Hold the bent elbow with your opposite hand and gently pull until you feel a slight stretch at the back of your arm and possibly also in the side of your upper back. Hold for 30 seconds.

3 Gently release and switch to the other side.

Ignore excuses and stay true to your goals

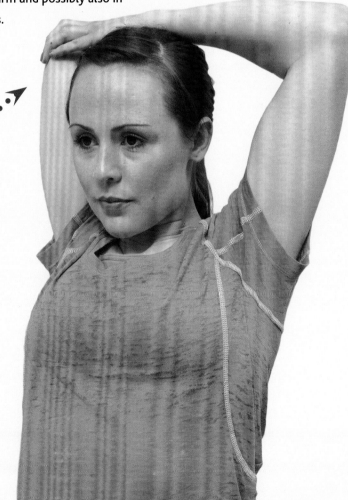

TIPS

Do not force your arm further than feels comfortable, you should feel a stretch, but not pain

The raised elbow should point upwards

Keep your head upright, neck in-line with spine

Breathe deeply and keep the shoulders and neck relaxed

cross shoulder stretch

This one is for the back of the arms as well as the shoulder muscles. This is an area where a lot of people hold tension and it can get very stiff and tight as a result. This stretch will help you to release that tension as well as minimising post-exercise muscle stiffness.

1 Stand up straight with your feet hip-width apart and your arms resting at your sides. Bend one arm to 90 degrees and raise it across your body at chest level.

2 Use your free arm to press the lifted arm in towards you, until you feel a mild stretch. You should feel the stretch mainly in the back of the shoulder. Maintain this position for 30 seconds. Switch arms and repeat.

3 Repeat again on the first arm, but this time keep the arm straight. Now you should feel the stretch more in the upper arm. Again, hold for 30 seconds per arm.

TIPS

Do not force the stretch, only press the lifted arm to the point where you feel the stretch

Breathe deeply and try to relax the muscles of the shoulders and arms as you press

Release the arm gently as you come out of the stretch

Keep your back straight and your head up

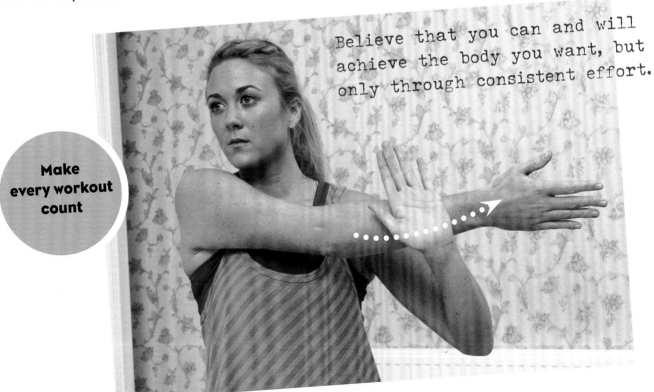

Believe that you can and will achieve the body you want, but only through consistent effort.

Make every workout count

wall pec stretch

This is a great stretch for the chest and shoulders, if you get a lot of tightness in those areas you're in for a treat – this is going to feel good!

1 Stand facing a wall. Extend your arm and place your right hand on the wall at shoulder level, with your fingers pointing out to the right.

2 Keeping your palm in place, turn your body away from the wall gently until you feel a slight stretch in your outer chest and shoulder muscles. Hold this position for 30 seconds.

3 Switch to the left side and repeat.

TIPS

Make sure your palm is flat against the wall.

Do not force the stretch – it may feel a little uncomfortable, but should never be painful

This is a static stretch so hold the position still

Your back should be straight, head upright

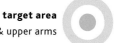

Exercise is nature's happy pill

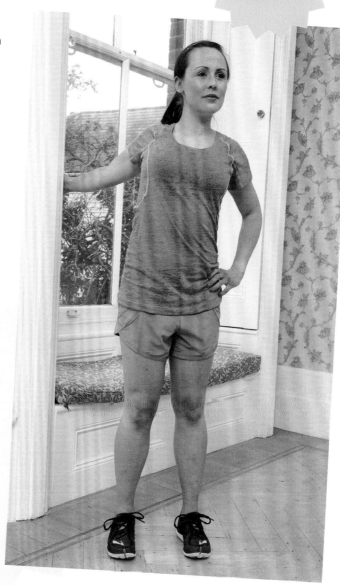

post-workout static stretches for the lower body

butterfly stretch

This yoga-inspired stretch is for the inner thighs and lower back. These muscles work hard in this programme and it's important to give them a little TLC.

Mornings are a great time to exercise — that way you get to feel smug all day!

1 Sit upright on the floor with your knees bent and the soles of your feet together. Take a deep breath, straighten the back and release as much tension as you can from your whole body as you exhale.

2 Place your hands on top of your feet and slowly lean forward from the hips until you feel the stretch.

3 If you're flexible in this stretch you can also gently press your knees downwards with your elbows, which will give you more of a stretch in the thighs. Hold this position for at least 30 seconds.

TIPS

Lean forward from the hips, keeping the back as straight as possible

Don't hunch your shoulders or tense your arms

Breathe deeply and stay relaxed

If this is uncomfortable for your knees, try moving your feet further away from your body

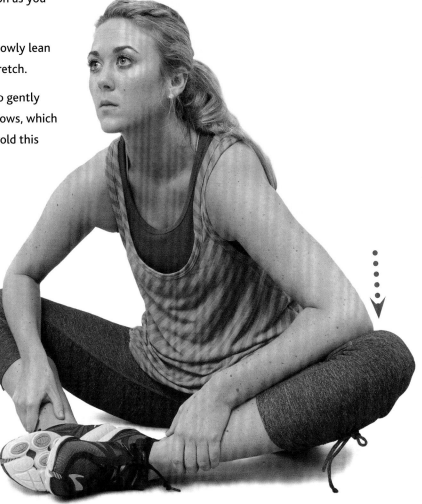

calf stretch

The calves work hard in a lot of the moves in the Fat Burn Revolution and could get tight and prone to cramps if not properly looked after. Here's a move that will help keep them happy.

1 Stand an arm's distance away from a wall. Take a big step forward with your right leg, keeping your left leg back. Extend your arms and slightly lean forward on the wall for support and balance.

2 Bend your right knee and press your left heel back down to the floor or until you feel the stretch in the left calf. Hold this position for 30 seconds. Repeat on the other leg.

3 Now take a shorter step back with your right leg and bend both knees. Allow your hips to drop toward the floor, but keep the pelvis tucked forward as you 'sit into' the stretch, feeling it lower down your calf. Hold this position for 30 seconds. Repeat with the left leg.

Keep thinking about your goals

TIPS

To increase the stretch step back further

Keep both feet and knees pointing forwards

Breathe deeply and relax as you hold the stretch

This is a static stretch so hold the position still

Keep your back straight at all times. Do not hunch over or round out your shoulders

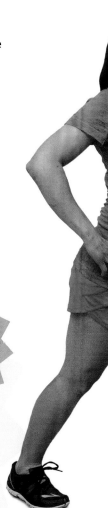
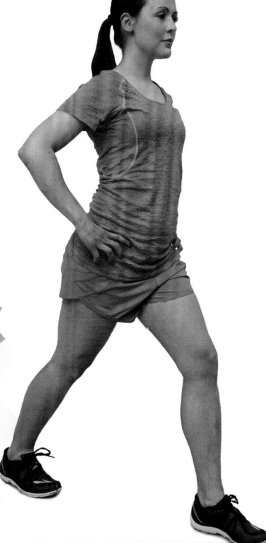

hamstring stretch

The hamstrings are large, powerful muscles running from the lower back down the back of the thigh to just below the knee. Tightness in this area is quite common among people who exercise regularly, so this is a very important stretch.

1 Sit on the floor with your legs together and extended straight out. Keep your back very straight.

2 Slowly bend forwards from the hips, pressing the chest down to the legs and extending your hands to reach for your toes. You should feel a mild stretch at the back of your thighs and lower back.

3 Maintain this position, gradually increasing the stretch until you feel mild discomfort. Hold this position for at least 30 seconds.

TIPS

Don't worry if you can't reach your toes, most people can't, just reach towards them. Hold onto your legs to pull yourself forwards if it helps

---

Increase the depth of the stretch gradually and slowly. Breathing deeply and relaxing into it will help

---

This is a static stretch so hold the position still

Keep your back straight, do not bend your spine to get further forward or hunch your shoulders

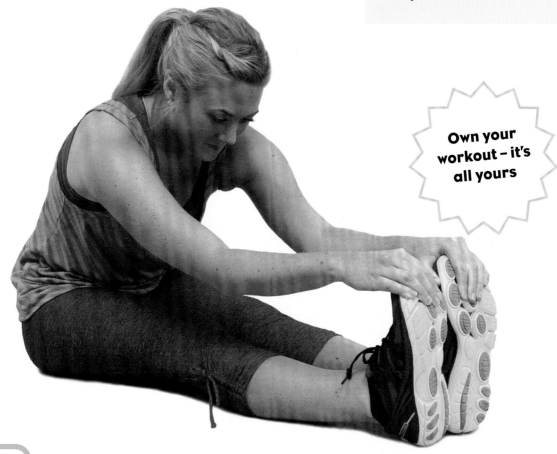

Own your workout – it's all yours

quadricep stretch

The quadriceps are large muscles on the front of the thighs that are key movers in the lower-body workouts. This move will reduce post-exercise soreness and help keep them flexible and loose.

1 Stand tall with your feet together alongside a sturdy object or wall to your left to hold onto for support if you need it.

2 Lift the right foot off the floor and, once you've found your balance, hold onto the heel with your right hand and gently pull the foot towards your buttock until you feel the stretch in the front of your thigh.

3 Keeping the back straight and not leaning forwards, hold the position for 30 seconds. Repeat on the left.

TIPS

Gradually pull the foot closer to the buttock to increase the stretch

To increase the stretch further, press your pelvis forwards

Keep the core muscles tight to help you maintain a straight posture

Breathe deeply and relax as you hold the position

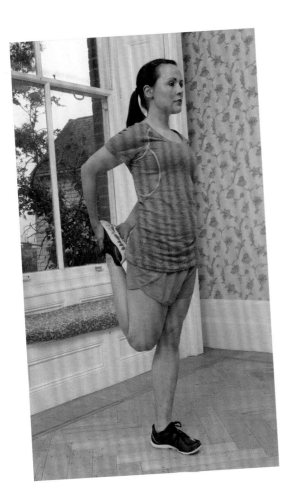

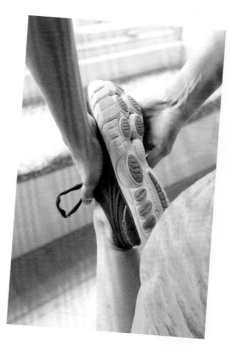

Look forward to that amazing 'I just smashed my workout' feeling you'll get when you finish.

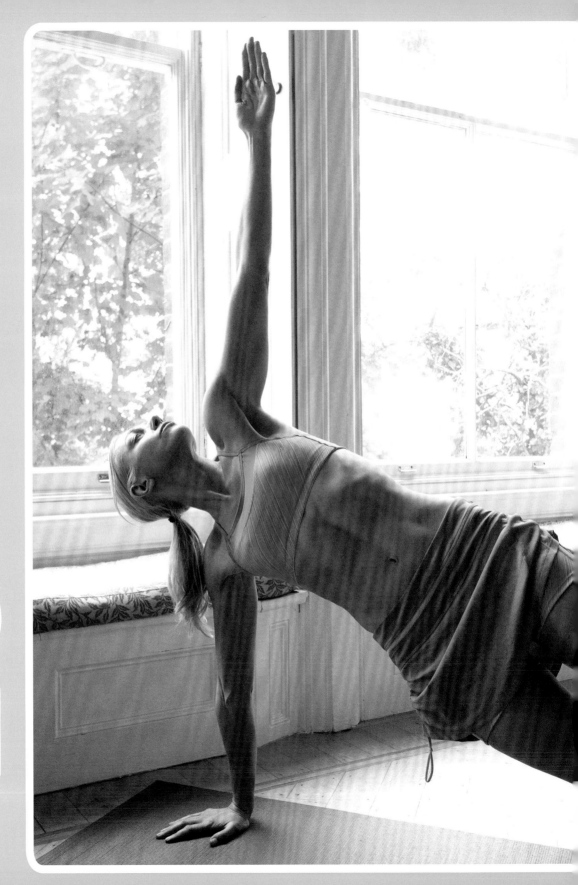

10 Phase I **workouts**

Phase I schedule

In Phase I you have two Metabolic Workouts, one which targets the upper body and one for the lower body, a Furnace Workout, and the Total Body Blast.

If you're new to this type of training, take it easy during the first week and focus on learning the moves, getting used to the combinations and the equipment, and building up the habit of exercising most days.

If you've been exercising regularly for a while and the moves are familiar to you then you should be able to dig-in from the start, but still go easy during the first week while you learn the structure of the workouts and find out what weights are right for you.

I suggest you schedule the workouts in this phase as follows:

On day seven, everyone should take a rest. Don't try to be a hero by training every day: that would be more likely to hinder than help your progress. To get the most out of the Fat Burn Revolution it's important to allow your body time to recover and adapt.

If you're a beginner or find yourself wiped out by day three, by all means take a rest. If you feel good, do the Body Blast workout. The same goes for day six – go with how you feel. But do try and get at least one Body Blast session in per week once you reach the third week of the programme. By this time your body will have started to adapt to this level of exercise by becoming a stronger, fitter, fat-burning machine!

day	workout
1	Metabolic Workout 1: Upper Body
2	Phase I Furnace Workout
3	Total Body Blast or rest
4	Metabolic Workout 2: Lower Body
5	Furnace Workout
6	Total Body Blast or rest
7	Rest

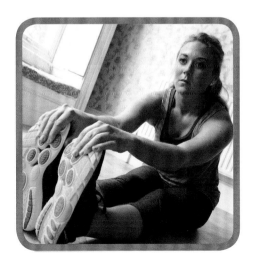

Phase I: Metabolic Workout 1 | upper body

As with all the Metabolic Workouts, use weights which you can only just manage to lift for the stated number of repetitions.

Each tri-combo is a group of three exercises performed one after another with no rest break between. Once you have completed all three you have earned a one-minute break. After those 60 seconds are up, repeat the three exercises once more before taking another one-minute break. Then move on to the next tri-combo.

You will probably find that you use heavier weights for the exercises in the first tri-combo than the second, this is simply because those exercises use larger muscles.

Use the rest period between the tri-combos to write down the weights used and number of repetitions you performed. If you manage the full number of reps with a weight then try increasing it next time. Remember, the heavier the weight, the more calories you'll burn while you're exercising and the more fat you'll burn afterwards while your body recovers.

Remember to warm up and perform the upper body dynamic stretches before starting and do the upper body static stretches at the end of your session.

tri-combo #1
- Bent-over row (p. 90) x 10
- Knee push-up or full push-up (p. 91) x 10
- Upright row (p. 92) x 10

1-minute rest

Repeat

1-minute rest and move onto tri-combo #2

tri-combo #2
- Shoulder press (p. 93) x 10
- Bicep curl (p. 94) x 10
- Tricep kickback (p. 95) x 10

1-minute rest

Repeat

1-minute rest and move onto tri-combo #3

tri-combo #3
- Superman (p. 96) x hold for 30 seconds per side
- Basic crunches (p. 97) x 20
- Side crunches (p. 98) x 20 per side

1-minute rest

Repeat

1-minute rest and perform cool-down

Phase I: Furnace Workout

In the Furnace Workouts you're going to exercise almost as hard as you possibly can, but only for very short periods of time. This means that you will push yourself much harder than if you needed to sustain the effort for longer because you know a break is only seconds away.

On a scale of effort where 1 is lying on the sofa watching TV and 10 is running for your life, you should be at 8–9/10 during the hard effort phase of the intervals.

During the warm-up phase, put in enough effort so you're at 6–7/10 on the effort scale. Do not begin the intervals until you're there.

If you're new to exercise or more used to long, slow, endurance type training you might find it difficult to push yourself to these levels of quick-burst effort at first. If these sessions seem at all easy, then this applies to you! Don't worry, after a few weeks you'll notice that you find another gear to use for this type of training.

interval structure

5-minute warm up

Begin performing your chosen activity at an easy, low intensity pace and gradually build up until you're at 6-7/10 effort over at least five minutes.

effort blasts

• Exercise at 8/10 for 30 seconds
• Exercise at an easy pace (around 3/10 effort) for 2 minutes

Repeat x 4

5-minute cool-down

Continue at an easy pace for five minutes while your heart rate comes down and breathing slows.

stretch

Stretch any muscles which feel tight or that you felt a burning sensation in during the session.

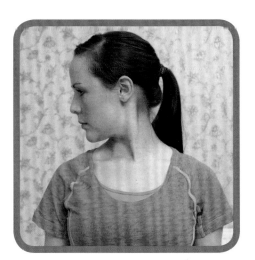

Phase I: Total Body Blast

This workout gets your whole body involved for super-fierce fat burning. No dumbbells/weights are required. However, if you would like to make it more challenging and super-effective it could be performed while wearing ankle weights.

There are six exercises, which you will perform for as many repetitions as you can for 30 seconds each. Once 30 seconds are up you take a one-minute break and record your number of repetitions before moving on to the next exercise. Once you have completed all six you have earned a one-minute break. After the break return to the first exercise and repeat the process again twice to make a total of three circuits.

Don't worry if you can't manage three circuits at first, just start with one and increase the number of the circuits as soon as you can. Once you have built up to doing three circuits, increase the amount of time you perform the moves to 60 seconds.

The faster the tempo on these exercises, the better the burn. Move as quickly as you can without losing form. It's OK to slow down if you get a bit wobbly, but do the best you can to keep fast and fierce and maximise the fat melt!

circuit

1 Knee push-up or full push-ups (p. 91) x 30 seconds
  1-minute rest

2 Steam engine (p. 99) x 30 seconds
  1-minute rest

3 Jumping jacks (p. 100) x 30 seconds
  1-minute rest

4 Plank (p. 101) x 30 seconds
  1-minute rest

5 Burpees (p. 102) x 30 seconds
  1-minute rest

6 Step-ups (p. 103) x 30 seconds
  1-minute rest

TIPS

If you don't have a sports watch, you might find an interval timer app of some kind helpful so you don't have to keep looking at a clock. People in the pilot group used various apps for various devices, visit juliabuckley.co.uk for links.

Phase I: Metabolic Workout 2 | lower body

This workout fires up some of the largest muscles in the body, which require a lot of energy to put into action – this means it has fantastic fat-burning potential if you give it your all.

These exercises can be done with no equipment, but the aim is to eventually do Supersets #1–3 while holding weights. You will perform sets of two different exercises back-to-back with no rest in between before taking a one-minute rest break. You will then repeat the two exercises twice, meaning you do each a total three times, before moving onto the next section of supersets.

Remember to warm up and perform the lower-body dynamic stretches before starting and do the lower-body static stretches at the end of your session.

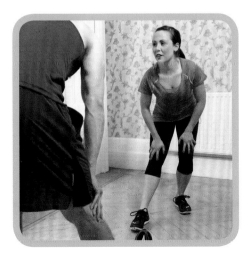

superset #1
- Forward lunge (p. 104) x 10 per leg
- Hip extension (p. 105) x 15

1-minute rest

Repeat x 2

1-minute rest and move onto Superset #2

superset #2
- Backward lunge (p. 106) x 10 per leg
- Leg lift back extension (p. 107) x 10
or good mornings (p. 108) x 10

1-minute rest

Repeat x 2

1-minute rest and move onto Superset #3

superset #3
- Squat (p. 109) x 10
- Calf raises (p. 110) x 10

1-minute rest

Repeat x 2

1-minute rest and move onto Superset #4

superset #4
- Lower ab leg lift (p. 111) x 10
- Arm lift back extension (p. 112) x 10
or cat (p. 113) x 10

1-minute rest

Repeat x 2

1-minute rest and perform cool-down

bent-over row

Bent-over rows provide an excellent workout for your upper back, plus they also hit the arms, core and legs. The benefits of this exercise include improvements in posture and a sexy svelte 'V-shape' in your upper back.

1 Hold a dumbbell in each hand. Plant your feet firmly into the floor about shoulder distance apart, bend your knees slightly then hinge forward from your hips, keeping your back straight and core muscles tight. Let your arms drop down towards the floor holding the dumbbells with palms facing your legs.

2 Squeezing your shoulder blades together, pull the dumbbells up to get towards your lower ribcage. Your upper arms should be at about a 45-degree angle to your body at the top of the movement.

3 Lower the weight back down in a slow and controlled motion to return to the starting position.

TIPS

Inhale as you lower the weights and exhale as you perform the pulling movement

Maintain a straight back and keep your neck in-line with your spine, so you'll be looking diagonally down to the floor in front of you

No jerky movements – perform the pull and release phases in a slow and controlled manner

Really concentrate on squeezing the muscles of the upper back to draw the weights in towards you

These are strong muscles, so make sure you pick up enough weight to challenge them

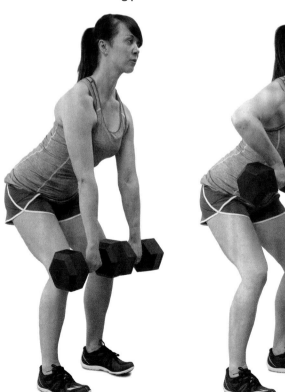

Every move takes you closer to your goal.

push-up

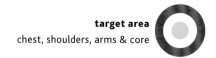

equipment
mat

The classic push-up is still widely considered one of the best exercises you can do. As well as shaping and firming your chest, arms and stomach, it helps improve posture and trains the body to move well as an integrated unit. The simplicity and effectiveness of this exercise makes it a brilliant choice for total beginners right through to the fittest of the fit.

1 Lie face down on your mat, legs together. Place your palms down on the mat at chest level, far enough apart so that your lower arms are perpendicular to the floor, elbows pointing directly upwards and aligned right over the wrists. Your upper arms should be at about a 45-degree angle to your body.

2 Beginners will be pivoting from bent knees with lower legs a few inches off the floor. If you're going for the toes, get up onto them. Keeping the whole body straight and rigid, push the palms into the floor as you straighten the arms and raise yourself upwards. This is one repetition.

3 Bend the elbows again and slowly lower the body back down as close to the mat as you can get, aiming to gently touch the mat with your chin before rising back up again.

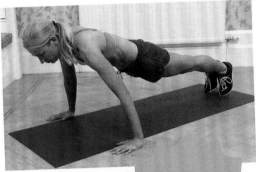

Know your limitations... And then defy them!

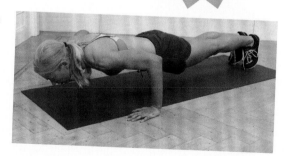

TIPS

Exhale gradually during the 'pushing up' movement, and inhale during the 'lowering' phase

Your body should form a straight line from head to knees or toes throughout the exercise

Take care to maintain that 45-degree angle with the arms – elbows should be lower than your shoulders

If you find the knee push-ups too easy, but still cannot perform them from your toes, try incline push-ups, which you do with your hands on a bench or some other sturdy object which will elevate you, making it easier than from the floor

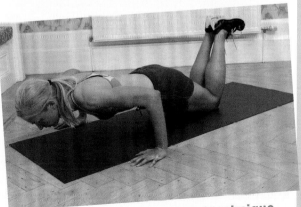

Advanced technique

upright row

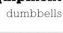

Upright rows are an excellent exercise to strengthen and shape your shoulders and upper back. If you're aiming to rock a halterneck or vest this summer, this is the move for you.

1 Stand in a straight and relaxed position with your feet hip-width apart. Hold your dumbbells in front of your thighs with your palms facing your body.

2 Keeping the dumbbells close together, pull both of them upwards until the upper arms are parallel to the floor and the wrists are just below the shoulders, allowing your wrists to flex as the dumbbell moves upwards.

3 Now lower the dumbbells back down in a slow and controlled manner back into the starting position and repeat.

TIPS

Exhale as you raise the dumbbells, inhale as you lower them

Maintain a straight back and keep your head up at all times

Do not pull the weights up in a jerky motion and control the movement as you lower them

If it feels uncomfortable to lift the weights to a point where your upper arms are parallel to the floor, either try a lower weight or just come up as high as you can if it is your flexibility which is limiting the movement (this will improve as you progress)

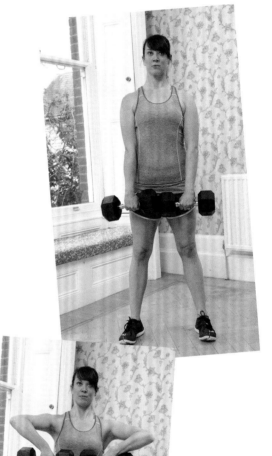

In this programme we don't exercise because we hate our bodies, but because we love them.

shoulder press

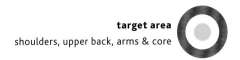

target area
shoulders, upper back, arms & core

equipment
dumbbells

Here's another well-proven classic exercise for the shoulders, upper back, and arms. This one offers fantastic aesthetic benefits – helping to shape, level and lift the shoulders and prevent slumping. The muscles activated in the shoulder press are important for every type of exercise as well as being key to everyday functional movements, so there are a lot of good reasons to give this exercise 100%!

1 Stand straight and proud with your feet shoulder-width apart, holding a dumbbell in each hand. Bend your elbows and lift both dumbbells to the sides of your shoulders, wrists directly above the elbows. This is your starting position.

2 Extend the arms above your head, pushing the dumbbells smoothly upwards, fully extending your elbows, bring the weights together at the top of the movement directly above your head.

3 Lower the dumbbells back down in a slow and controlled manner back to return to the starting position and begin your next repetition.

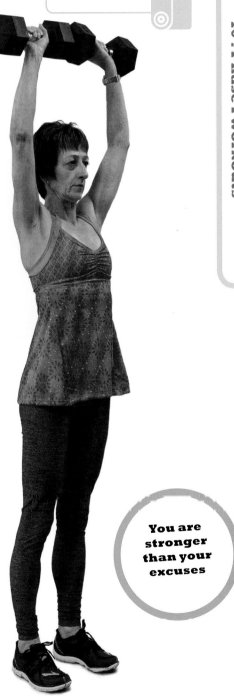

TIPS

Inhale as you lower the dumbbells and exhale as you press them overhead

Keep your back straight and aligned at all times and your core muscles engaged

Do not jerk the weights upwards or lock the elbows at the top of the movement

If you feel your grip on the dumbbells starting to fail or your arms get wobbly stop and complete your reps with a lighter weight

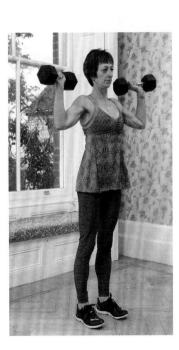

You are stronger than your excuses

bicep curl

Over the last few years, bicep curls have fallen out of favour in some circles, but I believe there's a good reason why this classic exercise has stood the test of time. They are simple and effective for firm, shapely upper arms, plus there's something very satisfying about mastering this old-school 'guns' move!

1 Stand tall with your feet hip-width apart. Hold a dumbbell in each hand, with the palms facing forward, arms down by your sides.

2 Raise both dumbbells by bending your elbows, 'curling' the weights up to your shoulders. Make sure that the inside of your upper arms stays next to your ribcage, do not let your elbows flare out as you lift. Concentrate on the bicep muscles on the front of our upper arms contracting and doing all the work.

3 Lower the dumbbells back down in a slow and controlled manner back, again ensuring that your elbows are still pressed closely to your sides. This is one repetition.

TIPS

Inhale as you lower the dumbbells and exhale when curling up

Keep the sides of your elbows pressed into your sides throughout the movement

Perform all stages of the movement in a slow and controlled manner

Keep your back straight, core tight and your head upright

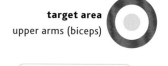

equipment
dumbbells

Take each session one exercise at time — you'll get through it, move-by-move.

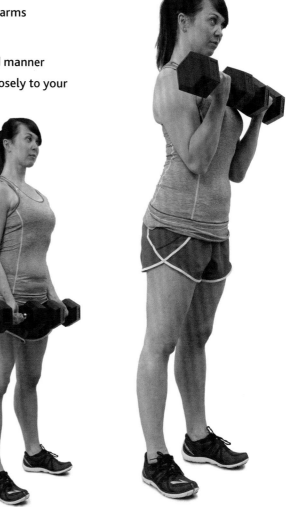

tricep kickback

If you want hard, chiselled upper arms, with that coveted definition on the back of the arm, this exercise is for you. It will isolate the tricep muscles to make them work extra hard, as well as hitting the core muscles which come into action to help you hold the position.

1. Start by standing tall with your feet shoulder-width apart. Hold your dumbbells with your palms facing your body. Bend your knees slightly and, keeping your back straight and core tight, hinge forward from your hips.

2. Keeping your upper arms tucked into your sides extend your lower arms backwards until your arms are straight and pointing diagonally down to the floor behind you.

3. Bring the lower arms back down to form a 90-degree angle with the upper arms before repeating the movement.

equipment
dumbbells

TIPS

Inhale as you lower the dumbbells, exhale when extending

Do not let the back arch or bend at any point

Keep your elbows pressed to your sides and concentrate on the back of the arms contracting and doing all the work

Keep your neck in-line with your spine, do not tilt your head up or down, you should be looking diagonally down at the floor in front of you

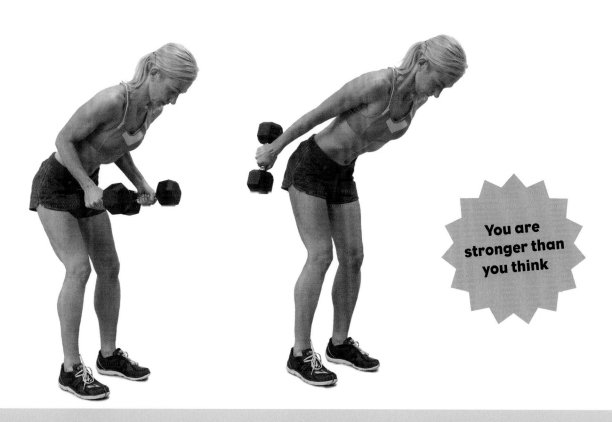

You are stronger than you think

Superman

You'll be down on your mat for this exercise working the lower back, core muscles and bum. Activating and strengthening these muscles will help you to move safely and efficiently, so exercises like this are very important foundation for real-world fitness. This is also a great exercise for improving posture and helping to correct imbalances in the way you move or stand.

target area
lower back, core & bum

equipment
mat

1 Get down on to your hands and knees. Knees should be directly below your hips and your palms on the mat with your wrists directly beneath your shoulders. Look down at the mat, keeping your neck in-line with your spine. Engage your core muscles and ensure your back is straight, not arching up or bowing downward.

2 In a slow and controlled motion, raise and extend your right arm until it is straight out beside your head, parallel to the floor. Once your right arm is in place, extend your left leg straight out behind you until it is also parallel to the floor. Hold this position for 30 seconds, maintaining a flat back and thinking about extending from your fingertips to your toes.

3 Lower the arm and leg back to the starting position then repeat with the left arm and right leg.

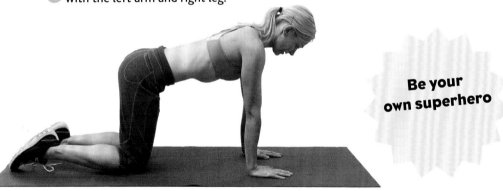

Be your own superhero

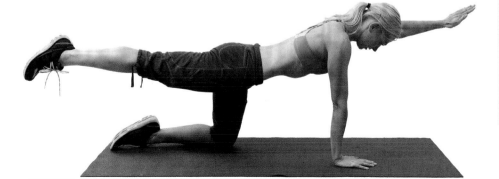

TIPS

If you're not used to core exercises this may be tricky at first so don't worry if you wobble, just attempting it will be giving those muscles a good workout

If you can't get your leg and/or arm parallel to the floor it doesn't matter, just raise them as high as you can. But you do always need to keep your back straight.

Control the movement as much as you can, don't jerk the arm and leg up and do not lift higher than parallel to the floor

Maintain control as you lower the arm and leg, slowly and deliberately returning to the start position

basic crunch

The abdominal crunch is a simple, easy-to-master tummy exercise suitable for even total beginners. Get ready to take your first step towards a flat, sculpted belly.

equipment
mat

1 Lie face up on your mat and bend your knees, placing the feet flat on the mat, close to your bum. Slide your hands behind your head to gently support the weight of the skull as you perform the exercise. Let your elbows point out to the sides and keep them in that position throughout the movement.

2 Exhale hard and pull in your abdominal muscles as you curl your ribcage and lift your shoulder blades up off the mat.

3 Hold for a second at the top of the movement and then gently lower your back down onto the mat. This is one repetition.

TIPS

Breathe out as you lift and inhale as you lower

Do not pull yourself up with your arms. Your hands are behind your head only to gently support the weight of it and take pressure off your neck

Keep the chin tucked in and do not jut the head forward, neck should stay in-line with spine

Do not let the elbows drift inward, concentrate on keep them pointing out to the sides

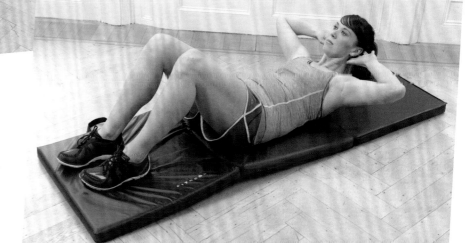

The only workouts you regret are the ones you fail to do.

side crunch

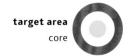

Side crunches are a simple yet challenging move to help tauten and tighten the sides of the waist.

1 Lie face up with both of your knees bent, feet flat on the mat. Twist the hips to drop your knees to one side, keeping your upper body flat on the mat. Place your hands behind your head in the same way as basic crunches.

2 Perform the crunch move by curling the upper body straight up off the floor, exhaling hard and contracting your abdominal muscles as you lift.

3 Pause for a second at the top of the movement before slowly lowering your back down onto the mat. This is one repetition. Complete your reps on one side before beginning the exercise on the opposite side.

TIPS

Breathe out when curling up and inhale as you lower

Use your hands to gently support your head, not to pull, let the abdominal muscles do all the work

Keep the neck and shoulders relaxed

Curl straight out in front of you, do not lean to either side

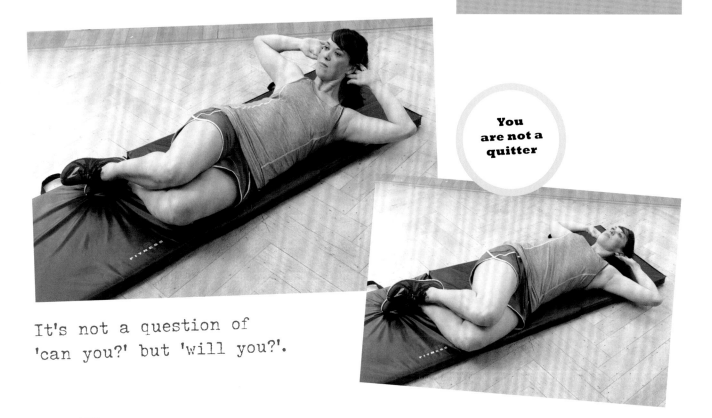

You
are not a
quitter

It's not a question of
'can you?' but 'will you?'.

steam engine

This exercise shifts your fat-burning engine into high gear and gets you puffing away like you're steam powered! You'll be building core strength, tightening the tummy and improving your balance in this locomotive-like move.

1 Stand up straight with your hands behind your head, elbows out to the sides, and your feet about hip-width apart, firmly planted on the floor.

2 Lift the left knee as high as you can while twisting the body down and bringing the right elbow down towards it. Aim to get elbow and knee to touch, but if you can't do that just press them towards each other as closely as you can.

3 Return to the starting position before lifting the right knee and lowering the left elbow. Keep repeating on alternate sides.

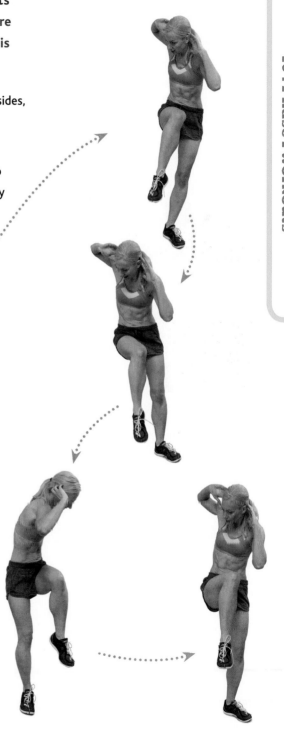

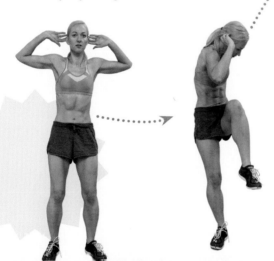

TIPS

Think about 'crunching' the abs as you bring the knee and elbow together

Exhale as the elbow and knee come in, inhale as you straighten up

Keep the elbows pointing out to the side of the head, do not allow them to creep in

Start performing the movement slowly while you master the form and then speed up the pace

jumping jack

Even if you've never been into exercise before starting this programme, I'm sure you're familiar with good old jumping jacks. It may look like kids' capers, but this exercise is a great quick-fire fat-burning move that jacks up the metabolic rate. These will also help prepare you for the plyometric exercises in Phase II.

1 Start with your feet together and your arms down by your sides. Slightly bend the knees and elbows and keep that 'softness' in the joints throughout the exercise.

2 Jump both feet out to a wide stance at the same time as raising the arms out to the sides and up above shoulder level, or to a point that feels comfortable.

3 Without pausing, quickly the jump the feet back in and return the arms to the sides. This is one Jumping Jack.

TIPS

Keep the back straight, core in tight and head up

If it doesn't feel comfortable to bring your arms up high, don't reach above shoulder level

Try inhaling for two jacks and exhaling for two if you have trouble regulating your breathing

Make sure you land on the balls of your feet to absorb the impact and protect the joints

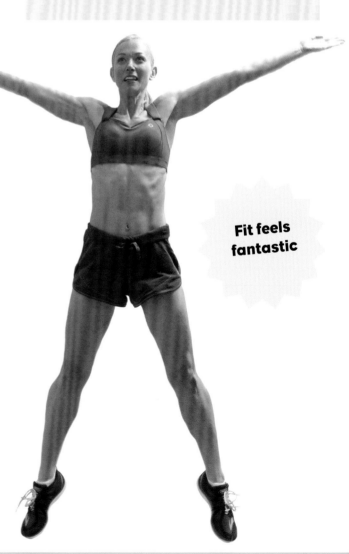

Fit feels fantastic

The more you exercise, the more you learn to love your body. It will never be perfect, but it will show that you are capable of doing more than you ever thought you could do.

plank

 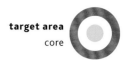
Planks are one of the best exercises for tightening the tummy because they work the whole midsection of your body, including the deep abdominal muscles. They are also great for improving posture and balance and will build core strength to help you perform better in all the exercises in the programme.

1 Lie face down on the mat. Keep your legs together straight out behind you and come up onto your elbows. Make sure the elbows are placed directly below the shoulders. Your hands can either stay palms down on the mat or you can clasp them together.

2 Keeping the back straight and head in-line with your spine, tuck your toes under and lift the hips and legs so that your body is now supported on your elbows and the balls of your feet. Your body should be in a straight line from head to heels.

3 Squeeze the buttocks and pull the tummy in tight as you hold the position. When you are ready to release, lower yourself slowly back on to the mat.

TIPS

If you're a beginner and can't manage the full plank, try doing them on your elbows and knees

Maintain a straight back and do not let your hips pop up or droop down

Do not hold your breath, you'll need to breathe from the top of your chest while contracting your abdominal muscles hard

Doing the plank in front of a mirror will help you achieve the correct posture

You
can and
you will

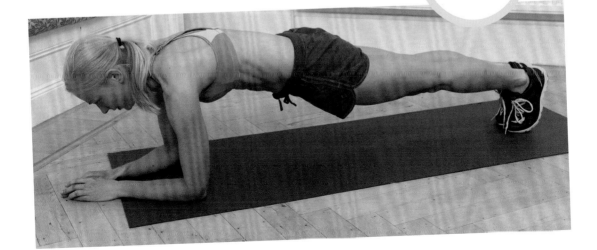

burpee

With its reputation as the exercise of choice of prisoners in solitary confinement, as well as being a favourite among the armed forces, the burpee is a bad-ass move that fires up all major muscles for a full body burn.

1 Stand with your feet facing forwards, shoulder-width apart, arms by your sides. Sit back into a squat, ensuring the knees track out over the feet. Lean forwards as you come further down and place the palms on the floor.

2 From this low squatting position, kick your legs out behind you, landing on the balls of your feet, to move into a plank position. Without pausing, thrust your knees back in towards your chest to return to the squatting position.

3 Raise your arms up above your head and jump up before returning to standing straight. This is one repetition.

TIPS

Correct form is very important. Remind yourself of the instructions for the plank and squat exercises before trying these

If you're a beginner, instead of jumping the legs out, you can start by stepping one leg back at a time to get from the squat to plank position and then stepping back in to return to the squat. You may also leave out the jump and simply rise back up to standing

Practise doing these slowly until you have mastered the move and then go as fast as you can while maintaining correct technique

To increase the intensity, add a push up before bringing the legs back in from the plank position

step-up

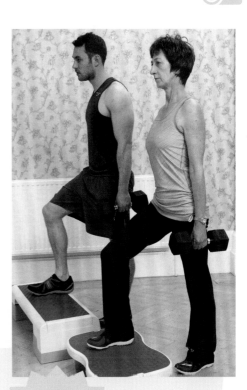

target area
legs & bum

equipment
step, bench or other
sturdy platform,
dumbbells (optional)

Step-ups are super-easy to master and offer fantastic fat-busting, thigh-firming, butt-lifting benefits! If you struggle with squats and lunges, step-ups improve strength and mobility in the same muscles that these two exercises employ, so to help you progress in these exercises, it's worth spending some time working on this move.

1 Stand tall in front of a step, bench or other sturdy platform with your hands at your sides, feet shoulder-width apart. If you're using dumbbells, just hold them down by your sides. Step up with your right leg making sure that your whole foot is firmly planted on the step.

2 Bring up your left foot and place it beside your right foot. Maintain a straight back and keep your head looking forward. Step down again with your right leg, followed by your left leg.

3 Instead of placing your left foot fully back down, tap the floor with ball of your foot before returning the left foot to the step, followed by the right. Repeat on the opposite side by returning the left foot to the floor and tapping down with the right before replacing the right foot on the step. Keep repeating on alternate sides.

This is about you vs. you

TIPS

Start by performing the exercise slowly until you get into a rhythm and then go as fast as you can while maintaining stability and a straight posture

To increase the intensity, after placing one foot on the step, raise the knee of the other leg up towards your chest and hold there for a second before placing that foot on the step

Once you have mastered this, add dumbbells for improved strength

Keep your back straight, head up and feet and knees point forwards at all times

forward lunge

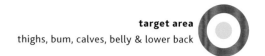
Perform lunges regularly with good form and you'll be rewarded with shapely thighs and a sexy firm bum. This move activates some very large muscles, which means your body burns a lot of fuel while doing them, so it's certainly a winner for fat loss. Plus lunges strengthen muscles that help protect the knees from injury, promote good movement patterns, and improve balance.

This could be one of the best moves you can do to ensure you stay mobile into later life. It won't be an easy exercise if it's a new one for you, but with all those benefits on offer, lunges are well worth mastering.

1 Stand tall with feet shoulder-width apart and take a long step directly out in front of you with the right leg, planting your heel down and then your toes as you move onto the ball of your left foot behind you. Allow your bodyweight to be supported equally by both feet. Take a few seconds to regain your balance if you need to.

2 Lower your body towards the floor, keeping your back straight, looking forward. Lower until your front thigh is parallel to the floor or to the point of discomfort (not pain). Don't worry if you find yourself leaning forward slightly (so long as you're not bending the back) but do try to keep the upper body as upright as you can. Ensure that your right knee does not flare out to either side, the shin should track forward over the foot.

3 Keep the front foot planted firmly on the floor as you use the front leg to push yourself back to the starting position and repeat.

TIPS

Breathe out as you lower into the lunge and exhale as you return to the start position

Keep your back upright and straight throughout the movement. If you wobble that's fine, just keep working towards maintaining your balance

If you experience pain doing this exercise, then stop immediately and consult a medical professional

Beginners have the option of placing a hand on a wall or sturdy object to keep steady as they learn the movement

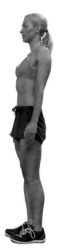
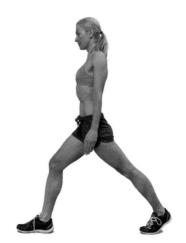
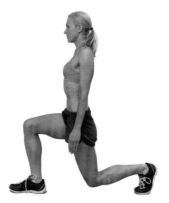

Think about the fat melting away

hip extension

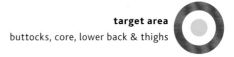
Hip extensions are a great exercise to lift and firm up the bum. They also offer the added benefit of working your core muscles, thighs and lower back. So these should help improve your posture as well as your posterior!

equipment
mat

1 Lie face up on your mat with your knees bent, feet flat on the floor. Keep your arms down by your sides – you can push down on the mat with your palms to help keep you stable as you lift if you need to.

2 Keeping your feet flat and your shoulders resting on the mat, gently lift your hips as high you can, squeezing your buttocks and keeping your core tight.

3 Hold the position for a second and then slowly lower the hips back down onto the mat. This is one repetition.

TIPS

Exhale as you lift the hips, inhale as you lower

Lift straight up, do not sway or tilt the hips and keep the knees and feet fixed in place

Lift high enough so that you feel tension in the muscles, but stay lower if it's painful to lift high

If you find this exercise easy, try doing it on one leg. Lift one foot off the floor and, keeping the knees together, extend the lifted leg straight as you raise the hips. Repeat on the opposite side

You are reshaping your body,
your lifestyle and yourself.

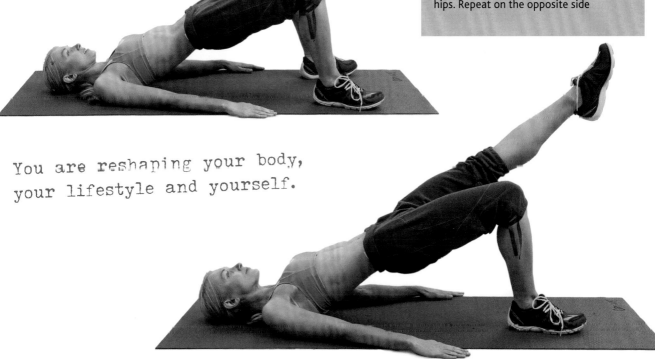

backward lunge

Here's another brilliant booty shaper! The backward lunge is a highly effective, easy-to-master exercise for firming and strengthening the front of the thighs and tightening up the bum. It also hits the core and lower back. Because it activates some large muscles, this exercise is a superb fat burner.

1 Stand up, straight and tall, with your feet under your hips, hands on your hips. Hold that upright posture in the back as you take a big step directly behind you with your right leg. You should now be balancing on the forefoot on the right side while your left foot remains flat on the floor.

2 Lower your hips towards the floor by bending the left knee, keeping your back straight, head facing forwards. Aim to get the left thigh parallel to the floor, but if you can't get down that low, just get as low as you can.

3 Press your front foot into the floor as you raise your hips back up. That is one repetition. Complete your reps on that side, step your right leg back so your feet are together again, then take a step back with the left leg and repeat on that side.

TIPS

Keep your back upright and straight throughout the movement. Do not sway to the side or tilt forwards

Both feet and knees should be pointing forwards, as should your hips

Short lunges target your thigh muscles a little more, while long lunges work your bum harder

Beginners may need to hold onto a wall or other sturdy object to keep steady during this exercise

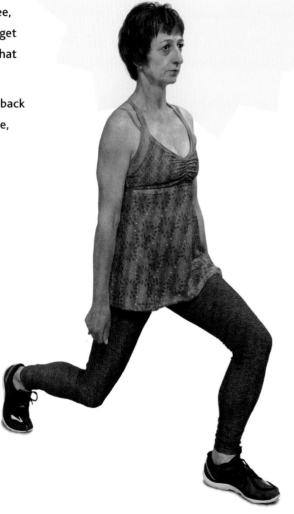

leg lift back extension

equipment
mat

Leg lift back extensions are the perfect complement to crunches as they work the muscles on the opposite side of the body. By targeting the muscles of the lower back they contribute to a well-balanced midsection and help improve posture, which also reduces the risk of back pain and injuries.

1 Lie face down on the mat with your arms crossed under your forehead and your feet and knees together.

2 Keeping your upper body still and relaxed, contract your buttocks and lower back muscles to lift the legs up off the mat.

3 After holding for a second, lower both legs to the floor in a slow and controlled manner. This is one repetition.

TIPS

Exhale as you raise the legs and inhale as you lower them

Keep your forehead on your hands and your upper body down on the mat

Don't worry if you can't lift your legs very high, so long as you can feel the contraction in your lower back you will be benefiting from this exercise. Keep practising and your range of movement will improve

Lift to a point that challenges your muscles, but is not painful

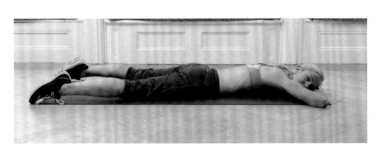

Dig in and feel it!

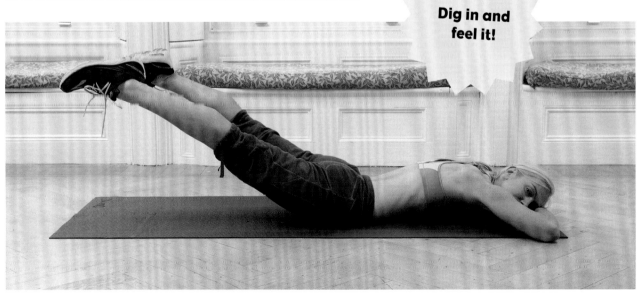

good morning

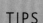

Performing good mornings will stretch out and strengthen the hamstring muscles which run from the lower back down the back of the thighs to the knees as well as improving core stability. If you find you get tightness in the hamstrings, this is going to feel great.

1 Stand with your feet hip-width apart, back straight and head up facing forwards. Place your hands on your hips.

2 Keeping your legs and back very straight, slowly hinge forward from the hips, coming down to the point where you feel a stretch in your thighs and/or lower back.

3 Maintaining a straight back, slowly raise your body back into the upright position. This is one repetition.

TIPS

Breathe out when lowering your torso and inhale as you lift

Maintain a straight back and legs throughout the movement

Place your hands behind your head to make it a little harder

Move in a very slow, controlled manner

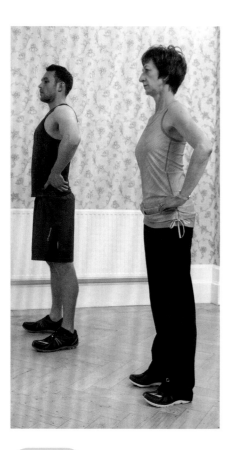

To make changes, you have to make changes.

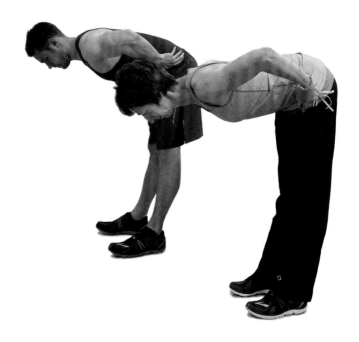

squat

target area
thighs, lower back, core, bum & calves

equipment
dumbbells (optional)

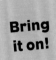

The squat is another exercise which is thoroughly deserving of its status as a time-tested classic. Squats are among the best exercises you can do for the legs and bum, and they also work the core and back muscles. They're a fantastic bodyweight-only move for beginners, or if you're more experienced you can up the ante by adding weights.

Bring it on!

1 Stand up tall with your feet shoulder-width apart. Beginners can start with hands on hips, or to make it a little harder, palms behind the head, elbows out. If you're more experienced hold a dumbbell in each hand.

2 Keeping your back straight, head up and core tight, bend your knees and lower the hips behind you as if you're sitting on a low chair. Make sure your feet stay flat on the floor and keep your knees aligned over the feet.

3 Aim to lower to the point where your thighs are parallel to the floor, or lower if your knees are comfortable. Push the feet into the floor and keep your knees aligned as you press the hips back up to return to the upright position.

TIPS

You should never feel pain in this exercise, if it hurts your knees then don't come down as low

Inhale as you squat down and breathe out as you raise yourself back up

It is very important to keep your back straight throughout the movement, a mirror may be helpful

Perfect the movement before adding weights

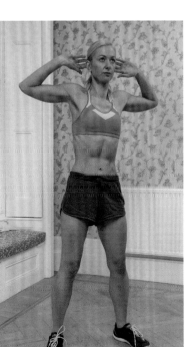

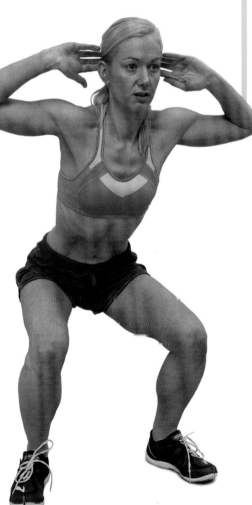

calf raise

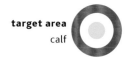

For sexy, shapely lower legs, this exercise is right on the money. Try them without weights if you're a **beginner** and once you've mastered the move you can add weights to work on getting that lusted-after heart-shaped definition in the back of the calf.

1 Stand tall with your feet pointing forwards, hip-width apart. If you're a beginner you might want to position yourself close to a wall or something sturdy to hold onto to help you balance.

2 Slowly rise up lifting the heels off the ground so you come onto the balls of your feet. Keep your legs straight and your feet and knees pointing forwards throughout the exercise.

3 Hold for a second at the top of the movement before slowly lowering your heels back down to the floor. This is one repetition.

TIPS

Breathe out as you lift your heels, inhale as you lower

Keep your back straight, hips tucked under and head facing forwards throughout the exercise

Once you have perfected the move add weights by holding a dumbbell in each hand

Another way to make the move harder is to perform it on one leg

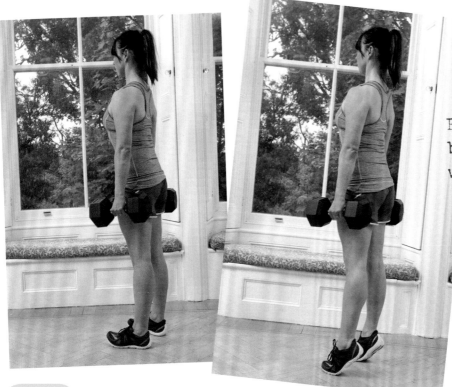

Each workout helps build new habits as well as muscles.

lower ab leg lift

Even people who regularly do exercises for the tummy often neglect the lower part of the abdominal muscles. Unfortunately this often results in their belly shape going to pot below the waist! Let's make sure that doesn't happen to you by smashing out some paunch-busting lower ab raises.

1 Lie face-up on the mat with both of your legs extended straight. You'll be keeping your knees and feet squeezed together throughout the exercise. Flatten your lower back into the mat and feel the contraction in your lower abdominals.

2 Without bending the knees, raise both of your legs, aiming to get them to a 90-degree angle to the floor.

3 Lower your legs slowly back down to the mat.

target area
belly

equipment
mat

TIPS

Exhale as you lift the legs, inhale as you lower them

Keep your hips and buttocks down on the mat, you are only lifting the legs

Perform the movement slowly with lots of control, do not swing the legs up or drop them down

If you cannot lift both legs together, lift one leg at a time, alternating sides to complete your repetitions

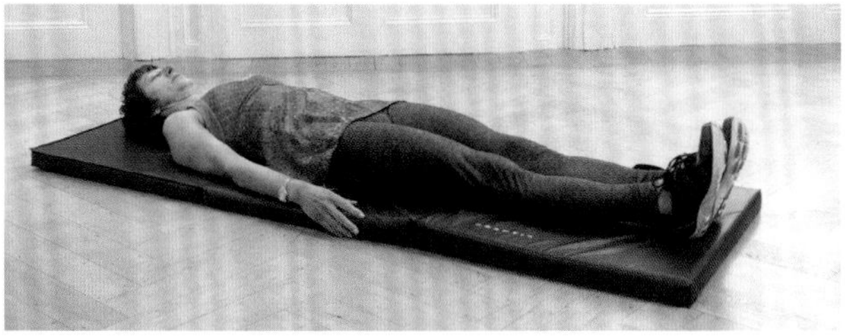

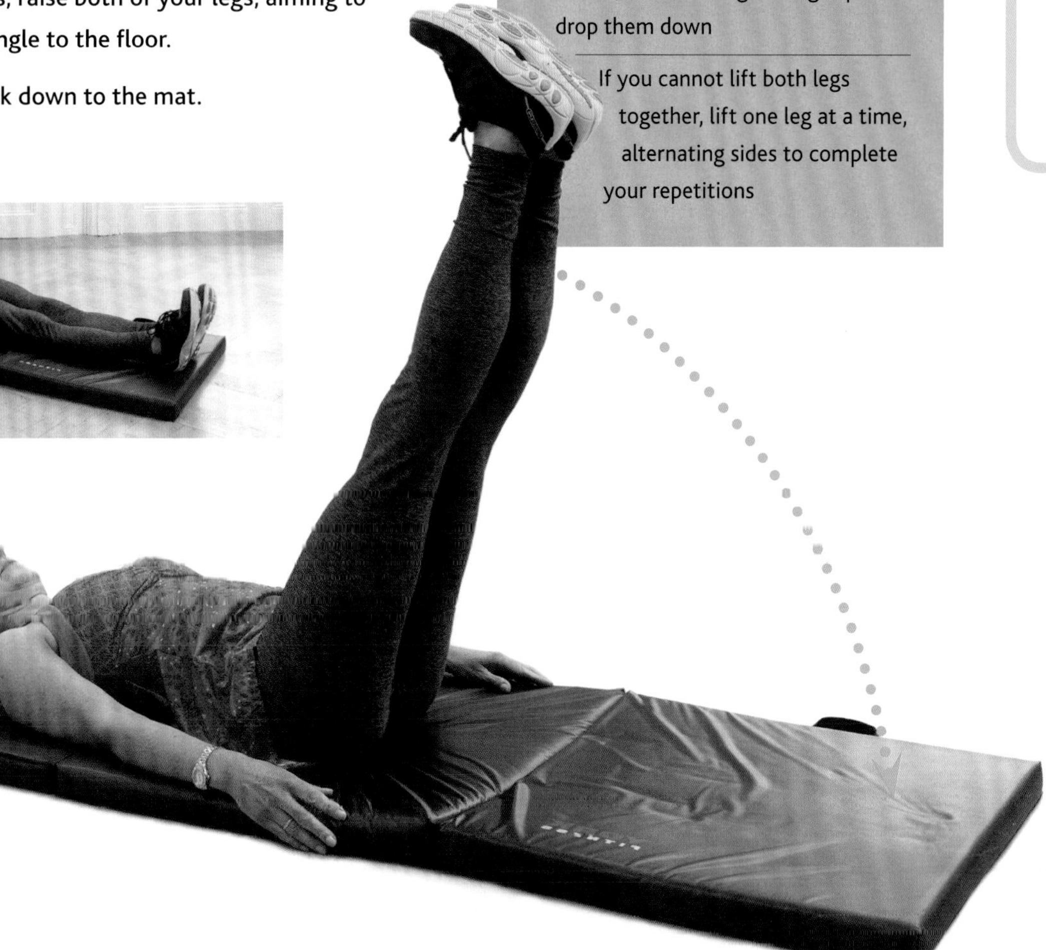

Say goodbye to the paunch

arm lift back extension

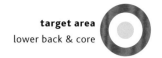

As with the leg lift back extension, this move partners well with abdominal crunches by targeting the muscles on the back midsection of the body to promote better posture, reduce injury risk and create a strong, shapely lower back.

1 Lie face down on your mat with both of your legs straight and pressed together. Extend your arms straight over your head, palms down.

2 Squeeze the muscles in your lower back as you raise your upper body off the mat in a slow and controlled movement. Keep your arms straight and in line with the body.

3 Hold for a second at the top of the movement before lowering your upper body gently, again in a slow, controlled motion back down onto the mat. This is one repetition.

TIPS

Breathe in when lifting your upper body and exhale as you lower

Allow the legs to relax and keep them flat on the mat

Don't worry if you can't lift your body very high, so long as you can feel the contraction in your lower back you will be benefiting from this exercise. Keep practising and your range of movement will improve

Lift to a point that challenges your muscles but is not painful

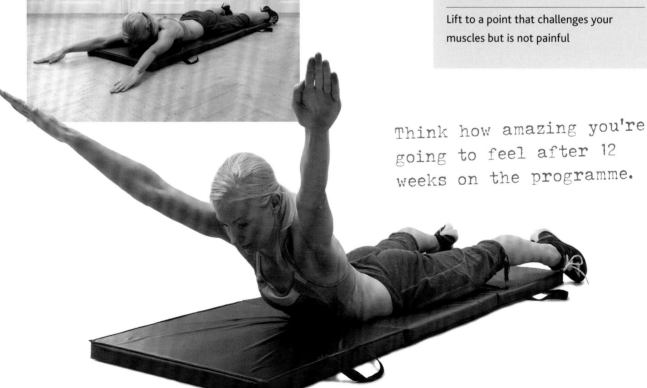

Think how amazing you're going to feel after 12 weeks on the programme.

cat

equipment
mat (optional)

The cat is an excellent exercise to loosen and strengthen the muscles around the spine. If you struggle with the back extension moves, this exercise should help you to perform those moves more comfortably. It also helps improve posture and tightens up the tummy muscles.

1 Position yourself on all fours with your palms on the mat directly underneath your shoulders and your knees underneath your hips. Keeping your neck in-line with your spine, look down at the floor.

2 Exhale hard as you pull in your abdomen and round your back up towards the ceiling, tilting your pelvis inwards. Hold this position for a few seconds pulling your tummy in as tight as you can and lifting your back as high as you can.

3 As you inhale, release your abs and slowly lower your back into the flat position and then down through to a downward arch, pressing your hips upwards. This is one repetition.

TIPS

It is important to work with the breath in this exercise: forcefully exhale as you lift and take a big inhale as you lower

Allow the abdominals to fully relax in the downward position

Move very slowly with full control

Work with your full range of movement, but do not push to the point of pain

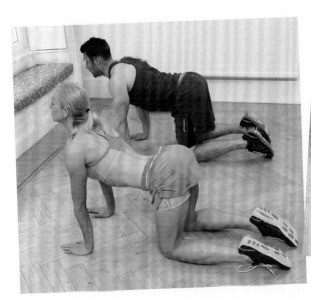

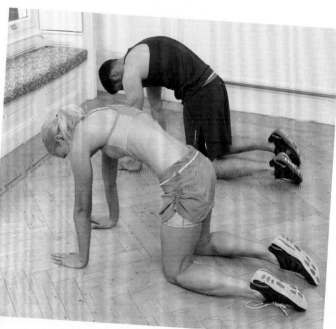

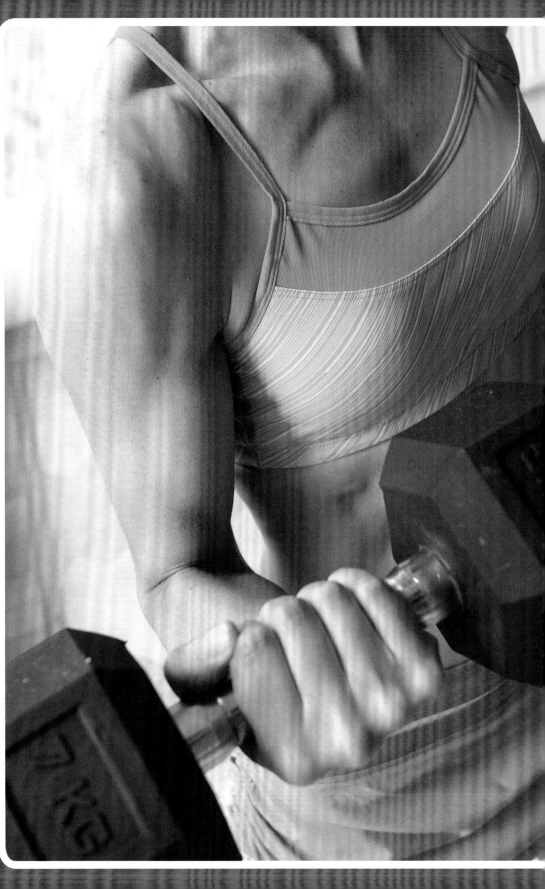

11

Phase II workout schedule

Welcome to Phase II of the Fat Burn Revolution fitness programme. It's time to ramp things up a little!

The training is going to get a little tougher, but the sessions are still short, fast-paced and varied.

You have four new workout sessions to do alongside your daily 30 minutes of steady paced activity which, as in Phase I, you need to do at least six hours before or after your workout of the day.

Please read all of the instructions on each of the workout sheets carefully before performing the sessions.

The standard weekly schedule for Phase II is:

day	workout
1	Metabolic Blaster – Chest & Back with Plyo Bursts
2	Metabolic Workout 1 – Legs, Bum & Core
3	Phase II Furnace **Workout**
4	Rest or Total Body Blast
5	Metabolic Workout 2 – Arms, Shoulders & Core
6	Phase II Furnace
7	Rest

If you're super-fit and keen to exercise six days per week you can insert the original Body Blaster workout on day four.

The Phase II Metabolic 1 and 2 workouts feature a warm-up set in each tri-combo. You should now be lifting heavier weights than when you first started the Fat Burn Revolution and some warm-up reps with lighter weights will help get the muscles activated and ready to work hard. As well as maximising performance and adding variety to the programme, the warm-up reps will reduce risk of injury, so do not miss this aspect of the sessions.

This phase has the potential to really accelerate your fat loss and fitness if you give it 100%. It is now even more important to eat a good wholesome diet to ensure your nutrition supports your fitness progress and fat-loss goals.

It's time to dig in, consistently follow the programme, forget excuses and really show your body that you're committed to the Fat Burn Revolution. Phase II is not easy, but definitely worth it. Enjoy!

Phase II: Metabolic Blaster | chest & back with plyo bursts

This session takes the metabolic workout to the next level. Alongside the muscle-building, metabolism-boosting resistance moves, each section features a plyometric exercise to develop explosive power and burn massive calories.

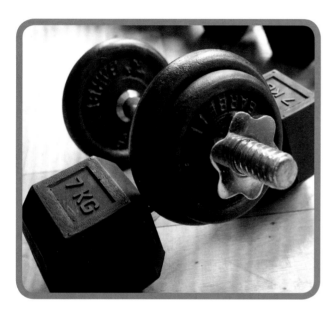

For the chest press, chest fly and particularly the dumbbell pullover (which involves passing the weight over your head), choose a weight that will NOT take you to the point of failure, but still presents a challenge.

format for each tri-combo

1 Perform each of the first two exercises with maximum weights or the most advanced version you can manage for the stated number of reps and then move on to the plyometric component without resting.

2 Perform the plyometric exercise for 1 minute or as long as you can – start by aiming for at least 30 seconds. If you choose an advanced version, you can regress to a less advanced version if you need to do that in order to complete the minute.

3 Take a 1-minute rest once you have completed all three exercises.

4 Perform your second set.

5 Take a 1-minute rest.

6 Move on to next tri-combo.

Remember to warm up and perform the upper body dynamic stretches before starting and do the upper body static stretches at the end of your session.

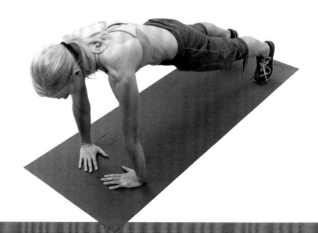

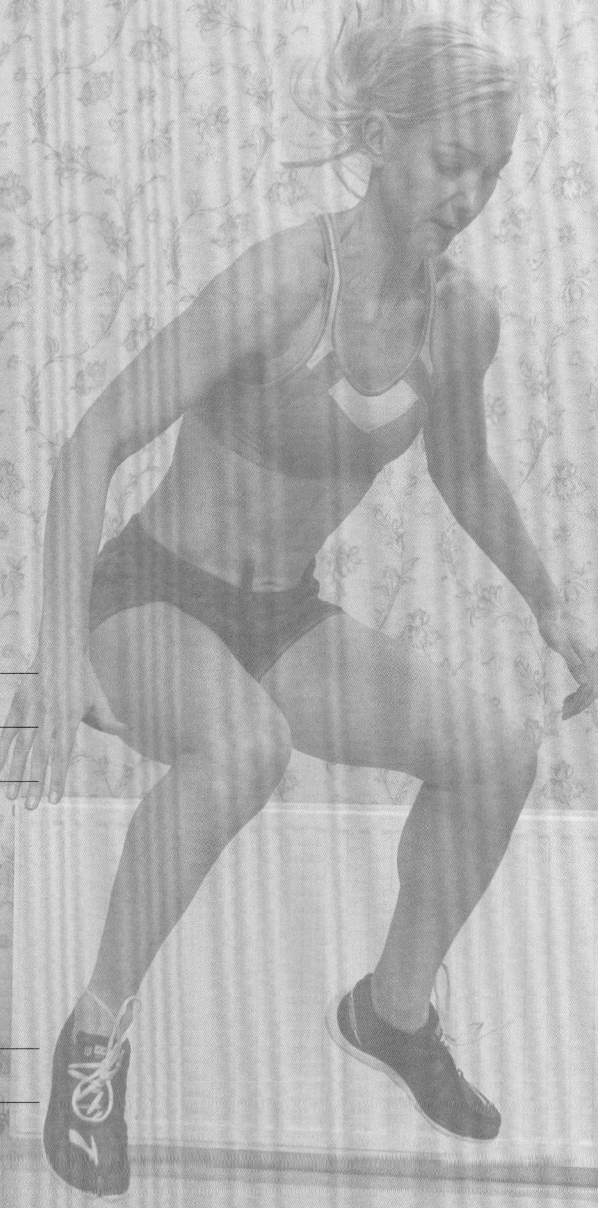

tri-combo #1

- Bent-over row (p. 90) x 10
- Dumbbell pullover (p. 125) x 10
- Jog in place with high knees – 1 minute

First full set then 1-minute rest

Second full set then 1-minute rest

Move on to next tri-combo

tri-combo #2

- Bent-over lateral raise (p. 124) x 10
- Chest fly (p. 125) x 10
- Burpees (p.102) – 1 minute

First full set then 1-minute rest

Second full set then 1-minute rest

Move on to next tri-combo

tri-combo #3

- Chest press (p. 126)x 10
- Close grip bent-over row (p. 127) x 10
- Jumping Jacks (p. 100) – 1 minute

First full set then 1-minute rest

Second full set then 1-minute rest

Move on to next tri-combo

tri-combo #4

- Standard push-ups (p. 91) x 15
- Airplane (p. 128) x 10 per side
- Box jumps (p. 129) – 1 minute

First full set then 1-minute rest

Second full set then 1-minute rest and perform cool-down

As always, the aim of the metabolic sessions is to push the limits of your strength and fitness, stimulating your body to make changes in order to adapt to new demands. This will help sculpt and define your shape, but most importantly it accelerates fat burning even when you are not exercising.

You should master the technique of these exercises before adding weights, but once you can do the stated number of repetitions while maintaining good form you can start adding some quite heavy weights as these moves employ the powerful muscles of the lower body. Because these muscles are large they require a lot of energy to fire up, which is great news for fat burning.

Weights are not required for the exercises using the ball or for the wall squat.

As well as the warm-up reps you still need to perform the upper-body dynamic stretches before starting and do the upper-body static stretches at the end of your session.

An intense workout is like a shower for the psyche; sweat out stress and finish clean

format for each tri-combo

1   Perform one warm-up set by doing each of the three exercises using a comfortable weight (around ¾ of your top weight) or the easiest version where weights are not used.
2   Take a 30-second rest
3   Perform your first full set by doing each of the three exercises with maximum weights or the most advanced version you can manage. Do the exercises consecutively with no rest between
4   Take 1-minute rest once you have completed all three exercises in the tri-combo
5   Perform your second set
6   Take 1-minute rest
7   Move on to next tri-combo

tri-combo #1
● Split squat (p. 130) x 10 per side
● Lateral lunge (p. 131) x 10 per side
● Gym ball hand-to-foot pass (p. 132) x 20

Warm-up set then 30-second rest

First full set then 1-minute rest

Second full set then 1-minute rest

Move on to next tri-combo

tri-combo #2

- Straight leg deadlift (p. 163) x 10
- Step-up (p. 103) x 10 per side
- Hip raise on ball (p. 134) x 15

Warm-up set then 30-second rest

First full set then 1-minute rest

Second full set then 1-minute rest

Move on to next tri-combo

tri-combo #3

- Forward lunge (p. 104) x 10 per side
- Wall squat (p. 137) – 30 seconds
- Back extension on ball (p. 133) x 15

Warm-up set then 30-second rest

First full set then 1-minute rest

Second full set then 1-minute rest

Move on to next tri-combo

tri-combo #4

- Ball leg curl (p. 135) x 10
- Squat (p. 109) x 10
- Gym ball plank (p. 136) – 1 minute

Warm-up set then 30-second rest

First full set then 1-minute rest

Second full set then cool-down and stretch

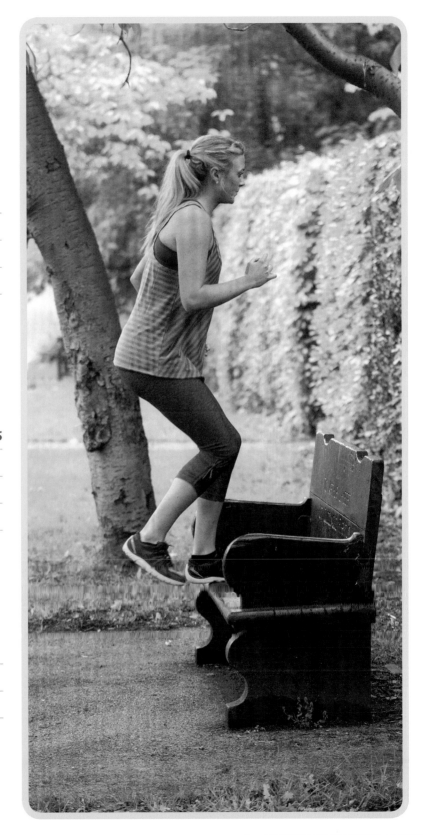

Phase II: Furnace Workout

This time you need to work a bit closer to your maximum level in the effort phase and you have a bit less time to recover between intervals. You'll also be doing six intervals rather than four. But now you've conquered Phase I, you're ready for this.

interval structure

5-minute warm-up
Begin performing your chosen activity at an easy, low-intensity pace and gradually build up until you're at 6–7/10 effort over at least five minutes.

effort blasts
- Exercise at 9/10 effort level for 30 seconds
- Exercise at an easy pace (around 3/10 effort) for 90 seconds

Repeat x 6

5-minute cool down
Continue at an easy pace for five minutes while your heart rate comes down and breathing slows.

Afterwards stretch any muscles that feel tight or where you felt a burning sensation during the session.

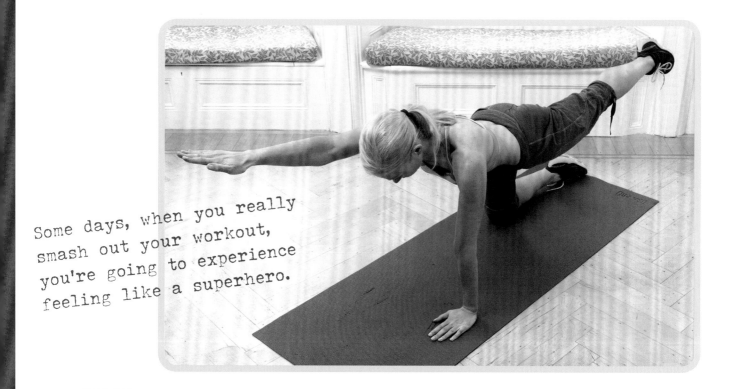

Some days, when you really smash out your workout, you're going to experience feeling like a superhero.

Phase II: Metabolic Workout 2 | arms, shoulders & core

For the core exercises which use weights – wood chop, Saxon side bend and Russian twist – it is not necessary to get to failure, but you should use a weight that presents a challenge for you in the stated number of reps.

In the case of exercises that do not require weights, perform the most advanced version of the exercise you can manage, even if that means you cannot complete the stated number of reps – just do as many as you can.

As well as the warm-up reps you still need to perform the lower-body dynamic stretches before starting and do the lower-body static stretches at the end of your session.

format for each tri-combo

1 Perform one warm-up set by doing each of the three exercises using a comfortable weight (around three-quarters of your top weight) or the easiest version where weights are not used

2 Take a 30-second rest

3 Perform your first full set by doing each of the three exercises with maximum weights or the most advanced version you can manage. Do the exercises consecutively with no rest between

4 Take 1-minute rest once you have completed all three exercises

5 Perform your second set

6 Take 1-minute rest

7 Move on to next tri-combo

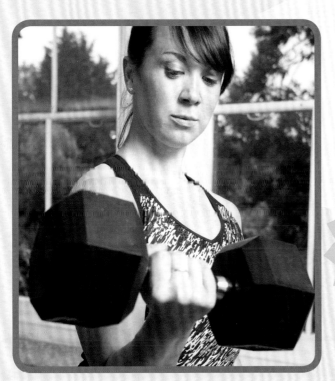

Fitter, stronger, leaner, healthier

tri-combo #1

- Lateral raise (p. 138) x 10
- Tricep push-up (p. 139) x 10
- Wood chop (p. 140) x 12 per side

Warm-up set then 30-second rest

First full set then 1-minute rest

Second full set then 1-minute rest

Move on to next tri-combo

tri-combo #2

- Single arm bicep curls (p. 141) x 10 per side
- Arnold press (p. 142) x 10
- Saxon side bend (p. 143) x 20 alternating sides

Warm-up set then 30-second rest

First full set then 1-minute rest

Second full set then 1-minute rest

Move on to next tri-combo

tri-combo #3

- Tricep dips (p. 144) x 10
- Diamond push-up (p. 145) x 10
- Russian twist (p. 146) x 20 alternating sides

Warm-up set then 30-second rest

First full set then 1-minute rest

Second full set then 1-minute rest

Move on to next tri-combo

tri-combo #4

- Upright row (p. 147) x 10
- Hammer curls (p. 148) x 10
- Palm-to-elbow plank (p. 149) x 20 alternating sides

Warm-up set then 30-second rest

First full set then 1-minute rest

Second full set then 1-minute rest and cool-down

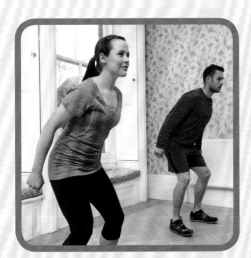

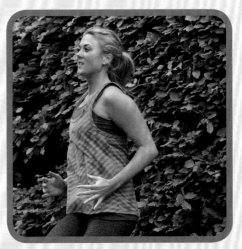

dumbbell pullover

The dumbbell pullover is something of a forgotten gem in my opinion. Not many people seem to include the move in their routine nowadays, which is a shame because it's a great 'value' exercise which works the entire upper body in a single swoop.

1 Lie face-up on a bench or flat on the floor with your knees bent. Firmly hold a dumbbell or single plate above your chest with both hands, straighten the arms, keeping just a slight bend in the elbow.

2 Keep the arms in position as you bring the dumbbell over your head and lower it towards the floor. Aim to get your upper arms level with your shoulders, but only go to a point that feels comfortable.

3 Keeping the back pressed into the mat or bench, raise the arms back up to the vertical position

target area
chest, arms, shoulders & upper back

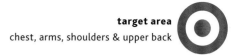

equipment
dumbbells, bench (optional)

TIPS

Exhale as your move the weight above your head, inhale as your return it to the start position

Keep your core tight and do not allow your back to arch up off the mat or bench

Maintain a slight bend in your elbows all throughout the movement

If you are on the floor, do not allow the weight to touch the floor (this will probably mean your arms don't quite get in-line with the shoulders, but that's OK)

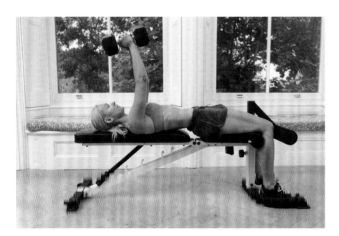

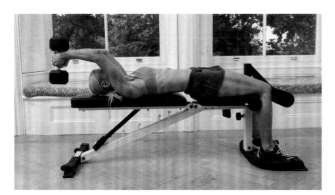

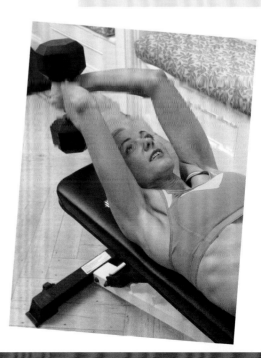

bent-over lateral raise

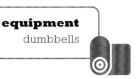

equipment
dumbbells

Not only is this exercise a superb shoulder shaper, it will also improve your posture, pulling the shoulders back for a prouder chest and athletic-looking silhouette. This is a good exercise to partner with the chest moves to ensure balance between the front and back of the body.

Strength can only be achieved by repeatedly challenging yourself.

1 Stand straight and tall, holding a dumbbell in each hand. Bend your knees slightly and, keeping the back straight, hinge the upper body forwards from the hips until your torso is almost parallel to the floor. Allow your hands to hang down towards the floor, palms facing each other holding the weights.

2 Think about squeezing the shoulder blades together as you raise your arms directly out to the sides, perpendicular to your torso, with a slight bend in the elbows. Make sure that your elbows stay higher than your wrists.

3 Slowly lower your arms back below you shoulders and repeat.

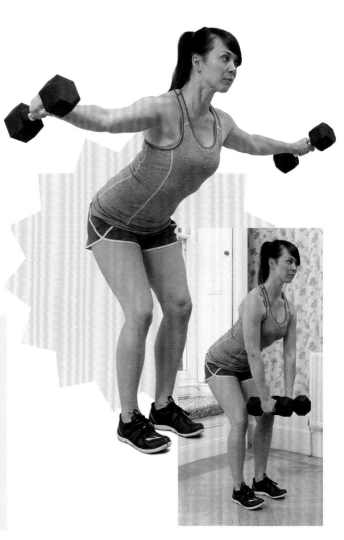

TIPS

Exhale as you lift the arms to the sides, inhale as you lower them

Keep the back straight, core tight and neck in-line with spine, you should be looking in front of you

Only raise the arms to a point that feels comfortable

Always keep your elbows higher than your wrists, it may help think about tilting your forearms slightly downward as if pouring water out of a jug

chest fly

Despite being a particularly tough move, this exercise is a favourite among many female fitness fans as you can really feel it in the pectoral muscles, which support the breasts, so you know you're helping to keep your assets lifted and firm! Guys love it too, of course – what man doesn't want perfect pecs?

1 Lie face up on your bench or on the floor with knees bent. Holding a dumbbell in each hand, with a slight bend in the elbows, extend the arms straight up above your chest bringing the dumbbells together, palms facing inwards.

2 Maintaining almost straight arms, slowly open the arms to the sides lowering the weights until they are at chest level.

3 In a continuous, controlled motion bring the weights back together over the chest, squeezing the chest muscles. This is one repetition.

target area
chest & shoulders

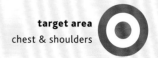

equipment
dumbbells, bench (optional)

TIPS

Inhale as you open the arms, exhale as you bring them back in

Do not let the arms drift down below the chest or up beyond the shoulders

Keep your back pressed firmly into the floor/ bench and do not allow it to arch up

Relax your neck and keep your head down on the floor/bench facing the ceiling

With commitment, perseverance and sweat, you will achieve your goals

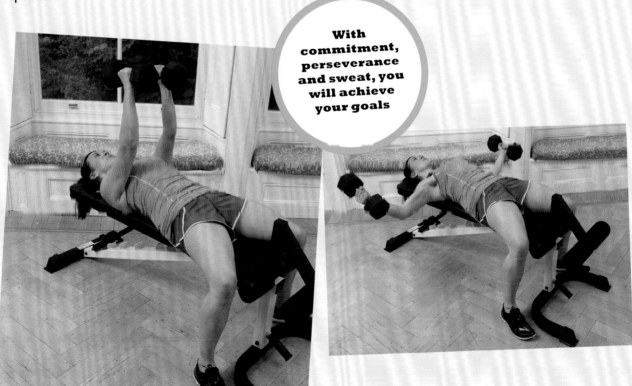

chest press

equipment
dumbbells, bench (optional)

Despite its macho reputation, the chest press is also a great exercise for the ladies as it firms the muscles which support the breasts, helping keep them firm and lifted. You may feel this one In the arms and shoulders too.

1 Lie face-up on the bench or flat on the floor with bent knees. Hold a dumbbell in each hand above your chest with an overhand grip, palms facing your toes. Keep your wrists in-line with the lower arms throughout the movement.

2 Bending both of your elbows directly out to the sides lower the dumbbells to chest level, or as low as is comfortable.

3 Push both arms back up, bringing the weights close together again above the chest in a slow, controlled arc.

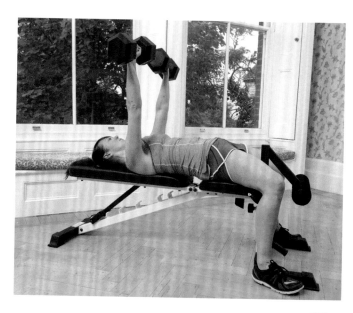

TIPS

Inhale as you lower the weights, exhale as you lift

Think about contracting the chest muscles as you lift and squeezing the shoulder blades together as you lower

Never bend your wrists, they should always be in-line with lower arms

The weights should move in an arc around the mid-chest level, do not let them drift up over the shoulders

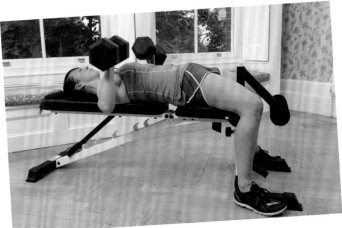

Strive for progress, not perfection.

close grip bent-over row

This exercise is very similar to the standard bent-over row from Phase I. By holding the dumbbells closer to your body you'll be working the muscles of the mid-back a little harder as well as firing up the biceps in the front of the upper arm.

1 Hold a dumbbell in each hand. Plant your feet firmly on the floor shoulder-width apart, bend your knees slightly then hinge the torso forward from hips, keeping your back straight and core muscles tight. Let your arms drop down towards the floor holding the dumbbells with palms facing your legs.

2 Bend the elbows towards the hips as you pull the weights in, brushing the sides of your ribcage with your arms as you lift.

3 Lower the weight back down in a slow and controlled motion to return to the starting position.

target area
back, arms & core

equipment
dumbbells

TIPS

Inhale as you lower the weights and exhale as you perform the pulling movement

Maintain a straight back and keep your neck in-line with your spine, you should be looking diagonally down to the floor in front of you

Lift and lower the weights in a slow and controlled manner

Keep the elbows in, do not allow them to flare out from the sides of the body in this type of row

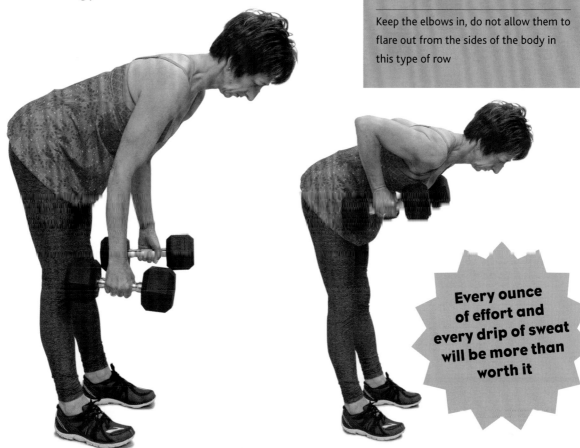

Every ounce of effort and every drip of sweat will be more than worth it

airplane

This move is awesome for fat burning because it activates lots of muscles, plus it helps firm the bum, strengthens the core and improves posture and balance. You may wobble or even take a tumble at first, so it's best to do these on a soft floor. Prepare for take off!

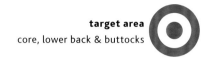

equipment
mat

1 Start on your hands and knees. Knees should be directly below your hips. Your palms should be on the mat with your wrists directly beneath your shoulders. Look down at the mat, keeping your neck in-line with your spine. Engage your core muscles and ensure your back is straight, not arching up or bowing downward.

2 In a slow and controlled motion, raise and extend your right arm until it is straight out beside your head, parallel to the floor. Once your right arm is in place, extend your left leg straight out behind you until that is also parallel to the floor – so that you are in the Superman position. After establishing your balance in this position, slowly bring your arm out to the side of your body level with the shoulder and your leg out to the opposite side as close to perpendicular to the body as you can get it without losing balance.

3 Return your arm and leg to the Superman position. This is one repetition. Do not return the arm and leg to the floor between reps. Once your reps are complete on side, switch to the other.

TIPS

This is a progress of the Superman exercise (p. 96), so only try it once you have mastered that move

Keep the core tight, taking shallow breaths from the top of the chest

Control the movement as much as you can, don't jerk the arm and leg up and do not lift higher than parallel to the floor

Maintain a straight back and tight core as you slowly move the leg and arm out to the side and back again

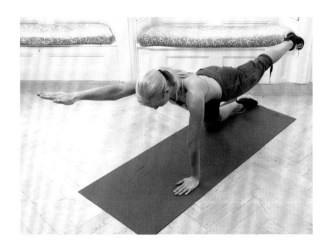

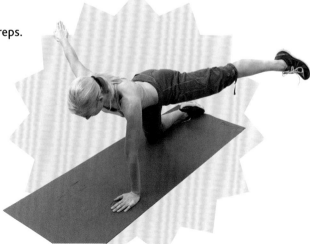

A strong core gives much more than awesome ab definition.

box jump

This is an intense, high impact move, which torches calories and builds explosive power in the legs. It's a tough exercise to perform, but has outstanding fat-burning potential.

target area
legs, bum & core

equipment
sturdy step or box

1 Stand with your feet shoulder-width apart in front of your step, head up, arms by your sides.

2 Bend your knees and lower your hips to prepare to jump. Make sure to keep your back straight and your head up at all times.

3 Power yourself up off the floor in an explosive movement as you jump up onto the step, keeping the knees bent as you land. To soften your landing, the mid-foot should land slightly before the heels come down.

4 Come back down from the box, either by stepping the feet down behind you, or if you really want to go for the burn, jump back down. Repeat without pausing.

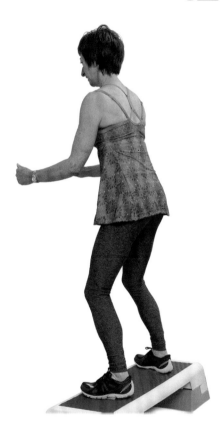

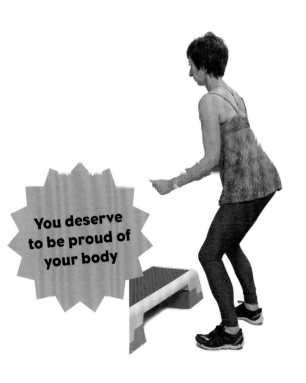

You deserve to be proud of your body

TIPS

This is an advanced plyometric exercise and it is only suitable for people with strong legs and healthy joints. If you have knee or hip problems or don't want to perform it for any reason, simply do the step-up move (p. 103) instead

Inhale as you prepare and exhale as you leap

Keep your back straight and flat, core tight and head up

Always land as softly as possible, with bent knees, hips back, mid-foot first

split squat

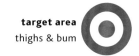

Split squats are similar to lunges, but most people find them a little easier to master because you don't step in-between repetitions. This means you can really concentrate on maintaining good form and giving the thighs and bum a great workout. In fact, this move works most of the muscles in the body and is a fantastic fat burner.

1 Stand straight and tall, with feet hip-width apart, toes facing forwards. Beginners should start with hands on hips and once you have mastered the move with perfect form you can raise the arms and place the hands behind the head, elbows out. When that becomes easy you can hold a dumbbell in each hand. Take a big step forward with your right leg. Come up onto the ball of your left foot.

2 Keeping your back straight, lower the hips towards the floor, bending both knees. Aim to get the front thigh parallel to the ground and a 90-degree angle in your left leg, but only go down as low as you can comfortably.

3 Push your front foot into the ground as you slowly raise your body back up. That is one repetition. Without stepping back in, complete your reps on that side before switching legs.

TIPS

Exhale as you lower, inhale as you lift

Keep your back straight and upright, resist leaning forward as you lower

You front foot should stay facing forward and remain firmly planted on the floor

Do not let you knees flare out or bow inwards

Refuse to give up on your goals

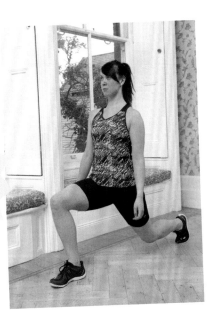

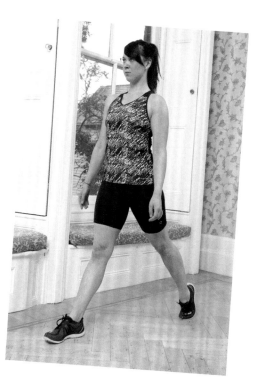

lateral lunge

target area
thighs & bum

equipment
dumbbells (optional)

Here's a move that targets the difficult-to-reach inner thighs. This one will shape and firm up those muscles as well as keeping that area flexible and supple. You'll also be hitting the outer thighs and buttocks.

1 Stand with your feet as wide apart as you comfortably manage. When you first try these just let your arms dangle by your sides. Once you're ready to add weights hold a dumbbell in each hand.

2 Bend your right knee as you push your hips out behind you, keep your back straight, head up. Aim to get your right thigh parallel to the floor, or as low as you can comfortably go. The left leg stays straight.

3 Press the right foot into the floor as you return to the starting position and repeat the movement on the opposite side.

TIPS

Exhale as you lower the hips to the side and inhale as your return to the centre

Keep the back straight and press the hips back as you lunge as if moving into a sitting position

Both feet should stay firmly planted flat on the floor at all times, pointing forwards or just slightly out to the side

Keep the knees in-line with feet, do not allow them to flare in or out

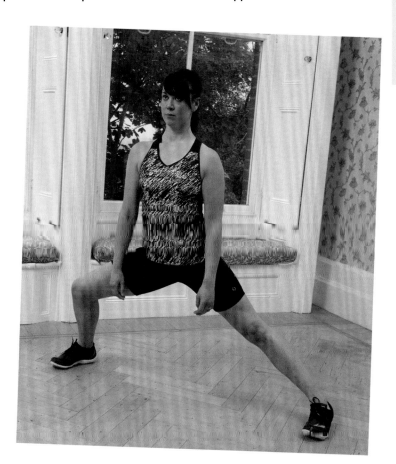

The challenge of this programme is as much mental as physical and you'll finish strong in mind and body.

gym ball hand-to-foot pass

If you dream of a flat, defined abdominal area, this move will take you several steps closer to making it a reality. It's a toughie, but incredibly effective – prepare to get shredded!

1 Lie flat on the floor, legs extended, holding the ball between your hands, arms outstretched over your head.

2 Keeping your arms and legs straight, lift them up and bring them together, raising the upper body as much as you can. Pass the ball from your hands to between your feet, squeezing the ankles together to hold it in place. Slowly lower the hands and feet back down.

3 Gently tap the floor with the arms and ball before raising back up again to pass the ball back to your hands. Lower again to tap the floor with your heels and the ball. That is one repetition.

equipment
gym ball

TIPS

Breathe out as you raise the arms and legs, inhale as you lower

Perform the movement slowly and with control

Keep the core engaged throughout, only briefly tap the floor between reps

The chin stays tucked in, neck in-line with spine

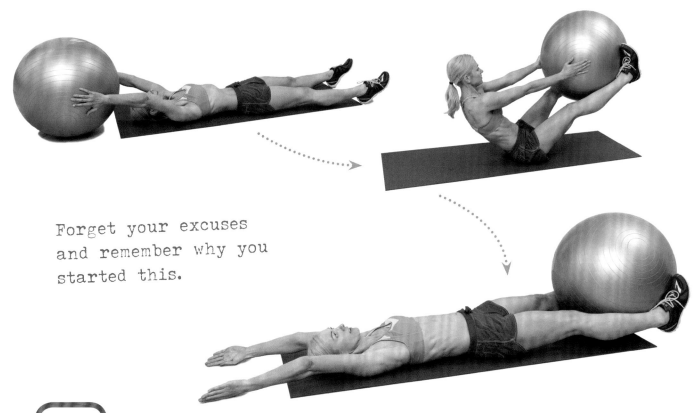

Forget your excuses
and remember why you
started this.

back extension on a ball

This is a progression of the back extension exercise from Phase I. Don't worry if you found you couldn't lift your body up very high, or at all, in the original version, you'll probably find that you can get more movement of the back in this version. By adding the ball you'll be increasing the range of motion as well as activating the stability muscles, you'll feel this in the buttocks a little more than in the original version too.

1 Hold the gym ball in place with your hands as you position your hips as close to the top of it as you can while still keeping your toes in contact with the floor. Beginners can have their feet against a wall to help keep the body in place. Your hands go behind your head, elbows out.

2 Contract the muscles of your buttocks and your lower back as you slowly raise your torso off the ball as high as you can go without discomfort. Hold this position for a second.

3 Lower your torso gently to the starting position and then repeat the movement.

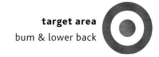

target area
bum & lower back

equipment
gym ball

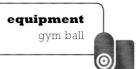

TIPS

Breathe out as you lift the body, inhale as you lower

Keep the neck in-line with the spine, chin tucked in. Do not lift or lower the head

If you're too wobbly in this position, try keeping the arms by your sides, palms on the ball

To increase the difficulty, extend the arms straight out so the upper arms are by your ears, fingers reaching forwards

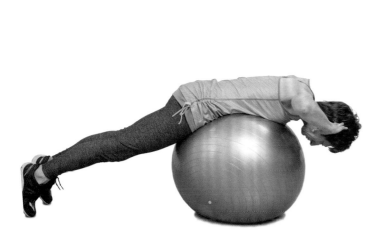

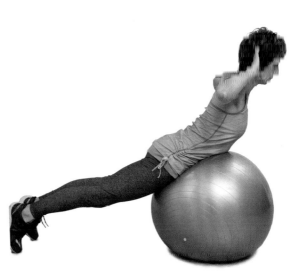

hip raise on ball

target area
core, bum & thighs

equipment
mat, gym ball

You'll love this one. You're going to flatten your tummy, firm up your thighs and buttocks and improve your stability in a single move. It is really a progression of the hip extension, which you learned in Phase I (p. 105), but this time you're going have your feet on an exercise ball. This is going to bring the muscles of your midsection into action much more as you'll need to hold them tight to perform the movement with good form. It will also mean the buttocks and thighs work harder to keep you stable and lift the hips that bit higher.

1 Lie flat on the floor and place your feet flat on the top of your gym ball. Your arms should be at your sides. You can press your palms down into the floor to help keep you stable when you first try this.

2 Brace the core muscles and squeeze the buttocks as you raise your hips until your body forms a straight line from knees to upper chest. Hold the position for a second, maintaining the contraction in your core and bum.

3 Slowly lower the body back down to the mat. This is one repetition.

TIPS

Breathe out as you lift the hips and inhale as you lower them

You can increase the difficulty by bringing your feet closer together

Keep the shoulders and neck relaxed. Do not lift your head

You may find it easier to do this exercise with bare feet

Motivation might have been what got you started, but perseverance is what will keep you going.

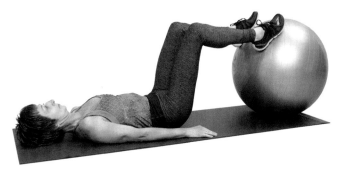

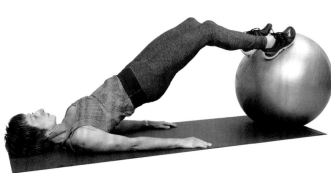

ball leg curl

target area
bum, thighs, core & lower back

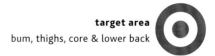

equipment
mat, gym ball

This is one of those exercises that might seem easy at first, but after a few reps, if you're doing it right, you should start to feel the burn. It's a great move for firming and shaping the back of thighs and it also hits the bum, core and lower back.

1 Lie face-up and place your feet on the ball. Keep your arms down by your sides, or if you're a beginner extend them out at a 45-degree angle and press the palms into the floor to help keep you stable.

2 Contract your buttocks, core and lower back muscles as you raise your hips until your knees form a straight line with your shoulders, as in the hip extension (p. 105). Now pull in your knees and roll the ball towards you, allowing your feet to roll on top of the ball. Aim to roll the ball as close as possible to your buttocks. Hold this position for a second.

3 Return to the starting position by slowly straightening the legs and allowing the ball to roll back under your feet. This is one repetition.

TIPS

Breathe out as you draw the ball in, inhale as you push it back

Keep your hips raised, do not return them to floor between reps

You can increase the difficulty by extending your arms over your head or for a really intense version, try using just one leg (switch sides halfway through your reps)

You may find it easier to perform this exercise with bare feet

Ready to play ball?

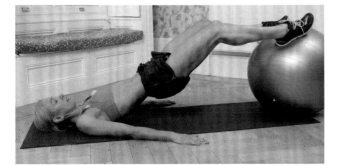

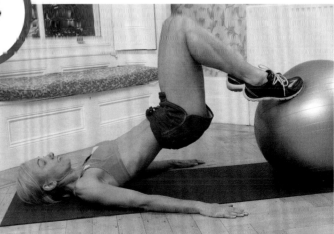

gym ball plank

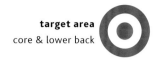

This is an amazing exercise for flattening and defining the stomach area. It's a progression of the plank exercise from Phase I (p. 101), but by placing the elbows on the ball you'll be forcing the core to work even harder as you fight the wobbles to hold the position. You'll also be strengthening the back and improving your ability to maintain good form in all standing exercises.

1 Kneel down in front of your gym ball. Rest your forearms on top of the ball, with your elbows directly under your shoulders.

2 Stretch out your legs behind you until your body is in a straight line from head to heels. Keep your feet together, you should be up on the balls of your feet. Concentrate on contracting the abdominals and squeezing the buttocks as you hold the position, aiming to stay as motionless as possible.

3 Slowly and gently drop the knees to the floor to release the position after holding for as long as you can.

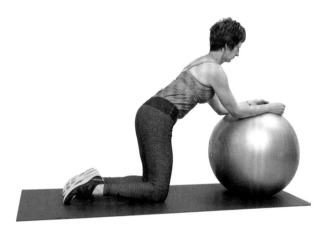

TIPS

Good breathing technique is key – think about taking breaths from the top of the chest to allow the abs to fully engage

Really engage the core in as you hold the position, imagine you're wearing a tight corset

Maintain that straight line through the body, do not allow your hips to drop or rise, keep the neck in-line with your spine

Don't let the chest creep forward, make sure the shoulders stay directly above the elbows

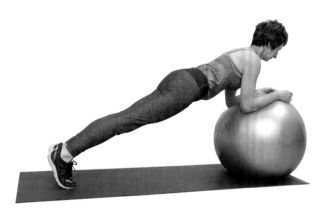

It's time to become the person you want to be.

wall squats

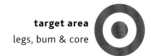

target area
legs, bum & core

This is a static exercise where you don't move at all – the challenge is simply to hold the position. But don't go thinking this is going to be easy, because it's not! Get ready to firm up the whole of your legs, your bum and strengthen your back, all without moving a muscle!

1 Stand up leaning your back against a wall. Slide your back down the wall, bending your knees until your thighs are parallel to the floor. Your back and hips should now be pressed firmly against the wall, your ankles should be under your knees, shoulder-width apart, feet and knees pointing forward, head up looking forward, arms relaxed by your sides. Make any adjustments you need to ensure that you have the correct position – you may need to shuffle your feet forward so that your ankles are directly under your knees.

2 Brace your core while you hold the posture as still as you can for as long as you can (up to a minute). Do not allow the knees to flare in or out, they should point forwards over the feet. When you can no longer hold the correct position it's time to come out of it.

3 Slide your body back up the wall to return to a standing position.

TIPS

Think about breathing from the top of the chest to allow the abs to fully engage

Keep the knees over the ankles and feet should be pointing forward at all times

Continually press the back into the wall

Allow the shoulders, neck and arms to relax

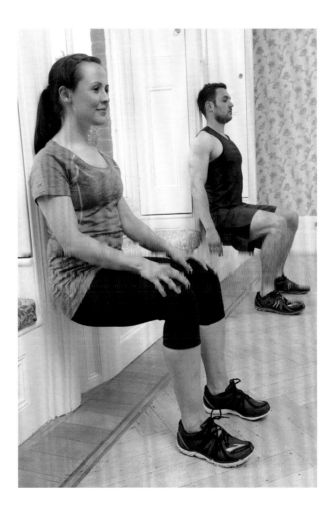

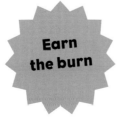

Earn the burn

lateral raise

If you want to look hot in sleeveless tops, this move is going to get you in business. The lateral raise is a great exercise for shaping and defining the outer shoulders as well as strengthening the upper back.

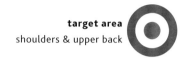

equipment
dumbbells

1 Stand straight and tall, feet hip-width apart. Hold a dumbbell in each hand, arms straight down by your sides, palms facing your sides.

2 Without bending the arms, raise the weights out to your sides to shoulder height.

3 Maintaining control, slowly lower the weights until they almost tap the sides of your thighs before repeating.

TIPS

Breathe out as you raise the weights, in as you lower

Do not lift the weights above shoulder height

Keep the back straight, head facing forwards, core tight

Beginners should start with very light weights

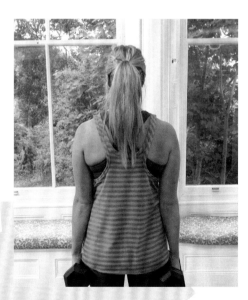

Will you throw in the towel or use it to wipe the sweat from your face?

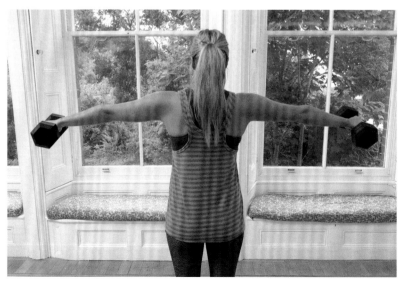

tricep push-up

equipment
mat

The tricep push-up is similar to the regular push-up, but with the hands spaced more closely together. This works the back of the arms to banish bingo wings and, as a bonus, it hits the middle part of the chest muscles more, to firm up the cleavage area.

1 Lie face down on the mat and place your palms down just below the shoulders so your elbows point to the ceiling and your arms are against your ribcage.

2 Come up on the balls of your feet or your knees. Push into the floor with your hands, keeping the elbows in, arms brushing the sides of the body until extended straight. As always in a push-up, your core should be tight and your body should form a straight line from head to heels (or knees if you are doing the beginner's version).

3 Slowly lower until your chin gently touches the mat, or as low as you can go, before repeating the movement. Again, make sure your elbows don't flare out, brushing the sides of your torso with your arms.

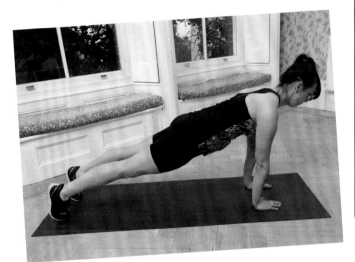

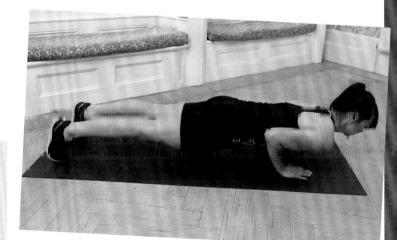

TIPS

Breathe out as you lift, inhale as you lower

Beginners should start on the knees, but get up on the toes as soon as you are able, even if you can only manage a few reps

Maintain a straight body and keep the neck in-line with the spine

Concentrate on keeping the elbows in, think about contracting the chest and back of the arms as you move

wood chop

This is a fun move to whittle your entire midsection, tightening the waist and improving the posture. Time to get your lumberjack on!

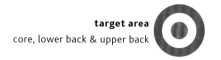

equipment
dumbbells

1 Stand tall with your feet shoulder-width apart, knees slightly bent. Hold a single dumbbell in both hands above your left shoulder as you prepare for the 'chopping' movement.

2 In a controlled motion, move weight across the front of your body. Lean forward slightly and rotate the torso as you bring the weight down past your right hip.

3 Raise the weight back up to the starting position and complete your repetitions on that side before switching the weight to the right shoulder and repeating on that side.

TIPS

Start slowly exercise then gradually build up speed

Keep your core tight throughout the exercise

Exhale as you lower the weight, inhale as you lift

Always maintain control as you move and keep a firm grip on the weight

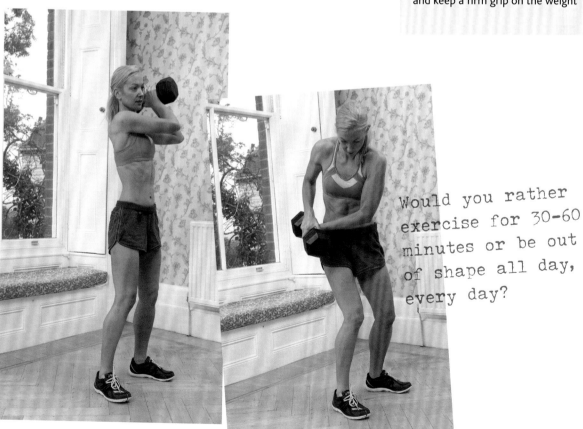

Would you rather exercise for 30-60 minutes or be out of shape all day, every day?

single arm bicep curl

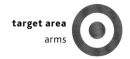

equipment
dumbbells

Time to work the guns! This is the same move as the bicep curl you did in Phase I (p. 94), but you'll be completing your reps on one arm at a time so you can really focus on good form and get the most out of this classic upper-arm defining exercise.

1 Stand straight and tall, head up, with your feet hip-width apart. Hold a dumbbell in one hand, arms by your sides, palms facing forwards.

2 Bend the right arm, keeping the elbow close to the waist and upper arm next to the ribcage, and curl the weight up to your shoulder.

3 Lower the dumbbell in a slow and controlled manner back into the starting position, making sure the arm stays tucked in. Complete your repetitions on the right before switching to the left arm.

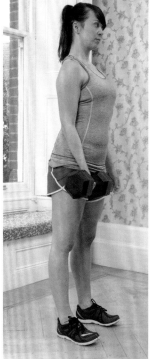

TIPS

Exhale as you lift the weight, inhale as you lower

Do not let your elbows or upper arms flare out or behind, keep them pressed close to your body as you curl. The other arm stays relaxed at your side

Control the movement, do not use momentum to swing the weight up or down

Maintain a straight back and keep the core tight

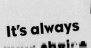

It's always your choice

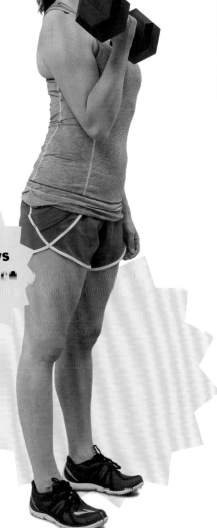

Arnold press

As you may have guessed, you can thank Arnold Schwarzenegger for this move. It's similar to the **shoulder press** exercise, but Arnie's version adds a flourish to engage more of the shoulder muscles and really sculpt that area.

1 Sit on a bench holding a dumbbell in each hand. Bring the weights up in front of shoulders, palms facing your body, elbows pointing to the floor

2 Open the arms to the sides keeping the elbows bent in the same position so your palms face forward and the weights are at the sides of the shoulders. From here, in a fluid, continuous motion, push the dumbbells up overhead as in the shoulder press exercise (p. 93).

3 In a slow and controlled manner, lower the weights back into the starting position in the same way, bringing them down to the sides of the shoulders and then together in front of you. This is one repetition.

target area
shoulders, arms & upper back

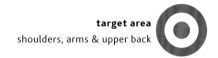

equipment
bench, dumbbells

TIPS

Exhale as you open the arms and raise the dumbbells, inhale as you lower and bring them in

Perform the exercise slowly, paying close attention to correct form and posture

You will probably need a lighter weight for this than you used for the standard shoulder press

If you feel your form starting to fail, stop and try a lighter weight if you wish to do more reps

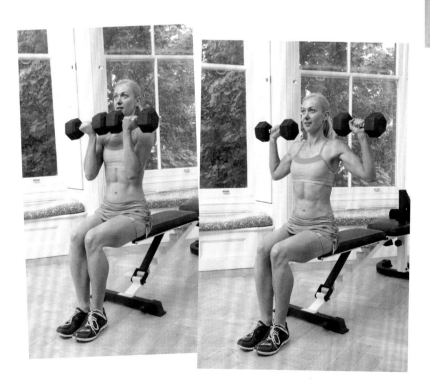

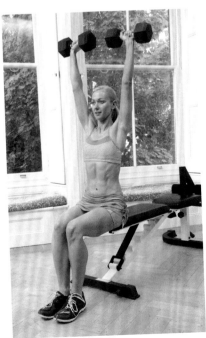

Saxon side bend

Here's a move to sculpt and strengthen your whole midsection. Be warned, it's harder than it looks, so try it with light weights to start with.

1 Stand straight and tall, feet shoulder-width apart. You can either hold a pair of dumbbells close together or a single weight with both hands. Raise the weight(s) up above your head until your arms are almost straight, just leaving a slight bend in the elbow. Palms should be facing forwards.

2 Holding the arms in position, bend your ribcage to the right using the muscles in the sides of your waist.

3 Return to the starting position and then bend to the left. That is one repetition.

target area
core

equipment
dumbbells

Be strong in body and mind

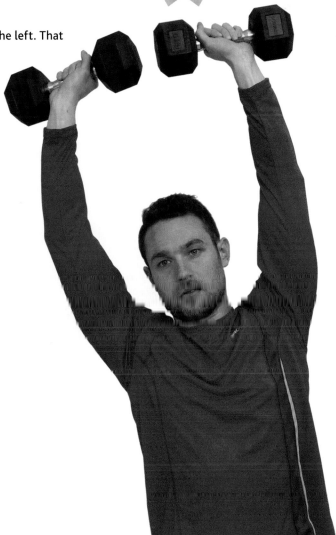

TIPS

Exhale as you bend to the side, inhale in the centre

Keep your back straight, neck in line with spine and try not to move the arms, all the movement should be coming from the waist

Move in a very slow, controlled manner

If it's too difficult with a dumbbell, try holding a bottle of water or even a cushion while you master the movement

tricep dips

This is one of my favourite exercises for firming and shaping the back of the upper arms. Master these and you can really start to tighten and define that tricky area. This move also benefits the shoulders, chest and upper back.

1 Start by sitting on the edge of your bench (or other stable object) and place your palms down onto the surface at either side of your hips, wrists facing behind you, fingers forwards. Your foot position will depend on how strong your tricep muscles are. Beginners can start with the knees bent, forming a 90-degree angle in the legs, and feet flat on the floor. As you get stronger move the feet further away until you are balancing on the heels with straight legs.

2 Grip the edge of your bench with your hands as you straighten your elbows and lift the body so your weight is supported on your arms. Lower your body towards the floor in front of the bench. Keep the hips and back close to the bench and the elbows pointing straight out behind you. Aim to come down until your upper arms are parallel to the floor.

3 Once your reach the bottom of the movement, push through the hands and straighten the arms to raise your body back up and repeat. Keep the hips in front of the bench, do not return to sitting between reps.

TIPS

Inhale when lowering your body and exhale hard when pushing up

Maintain a slight bend in your elbows at all times to keep your triceps engaged

Your elbows should always be pointing straight out behind you, arms tucked closely to your sides, do not allow them to flare in or out

Move in a slow and controlled motion, maintaining the same speed for lowering and raising the body

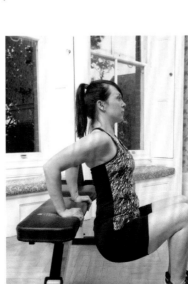

Your body might be complaining now, but it'll thank you later!

diamond push-up

Want well-shaped arms and a firm lifted chest? Be your own 'breast' friend and do some delectable diamond push-ups. It's not an easy move, but the results rock!

1 Kneel down then lean forwards, placing your palms down on the mat. Touch the tips of your thumbs and first fingers together to form a diamond shape between your hands. Point your elbows out to the sides to form another diamond shape. If you are a beginner, move your hands a few inches apart (the further apart you move the hands, the easier it will be). Beginners can also start out performing the move from the knees as with the stand and push-up (p. 91).

2 Without moving the palms, push into the mat as you straighten the arms. As usual with push-up exercises, at the top of the movement your body should form a straight line from head to heels.

3 Bending the elbows out to the sides once more, slowly lower yourself back down until the chest is as close to the hands (without touching) as you can get it. That is one repetition.

target area
chest, shoulders, arms & core

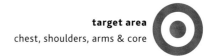

equipment
mat

TIPS

Breathe out as you lift the body, inhale as you lower

Maintain a straight body and keep your core tight at all times

Lower and raise your body slowly and with control

Keep the elbows pointing directly out to the sides and palms down with fingers and thumbs pointing diagonally towards each other

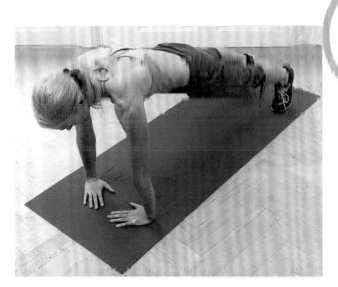

Think about pushing away all doubts

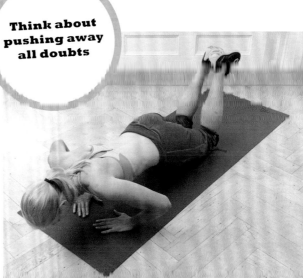

Russian twist

This is a satisfying move as you can really feel the deep core muscles working to squeeze in the waist and firm up the belly. Concentrate on keeping the back and legs as straight as you can for maximum results.

1 Beginners should start doing this without a weight – just clasp the hands together. Once you've mastered the move you can hold a single dumbbell or weight plate in both hands. Sit upright with your knees bent and your feet flat on the mat. Raise your hands/weight up to eye level and lean back a little as lift your feet up, so you're balancing on your bum.

2 Keeping the core tight, bring the hands/weight down to the right side to tap the mat.

3 Without pausing, lift the hands/weight back up to eye level and across down to the left side. This is one repetition.

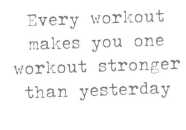

equipment
mat, dumbbells (optional)

TIPS

Breathe out as you lower the weight, inhale as you return it to the centre

Extending your legs will add intensity, keep them as straight as you can while maintaining good form

Keep your tummy tight and back straight at all times

Control the movement, do not swing the weight to either side

Every workout
makes you one
workout stronger
than yesterday

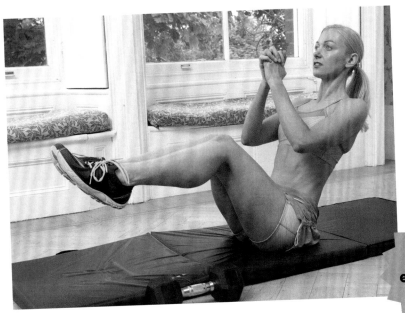

**Relish
every rep**

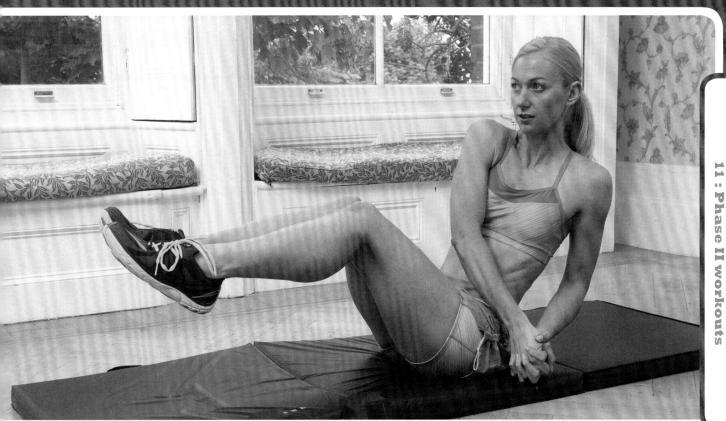

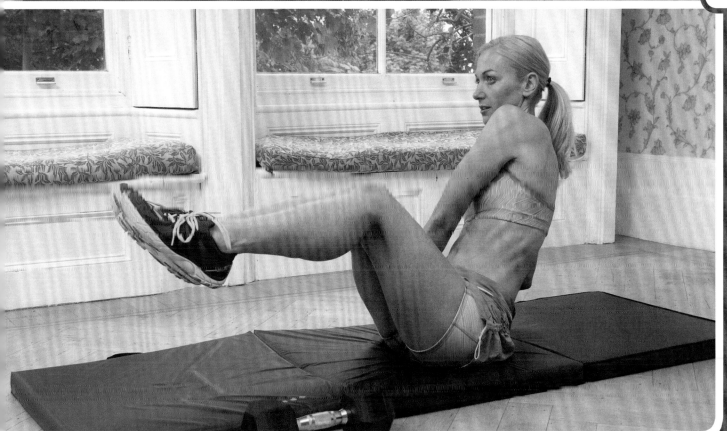

hammer curl

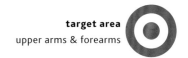

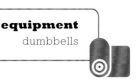

Hammer curls are another variation of the classic bicep curls, you'll still be mainly shaping the upper arms, but you'll also be strengthening and sculpting the lower arms a little more this time due to the different hand position. These also help improve grip strength, which becomes important as you move onto more advanced exercises.

1 Stand straight and tall with your feet hip-width apart. Grab a dumbbell in each hand and start with your arms at your sides with the palms facing your sides.

2 Curl both dumbbells up at the same time, bending at the elbows and bringing the weights up to the shoulders. Maintain the 'hammer' position with palms facing each other and do not twist the wrists or forearms. Keep your forearms pressed into your sides.

3 Slowly lower the dumbbells back to the starting position. That is one repetition

The feeling of achievement that comes with improved fitness is priceless.

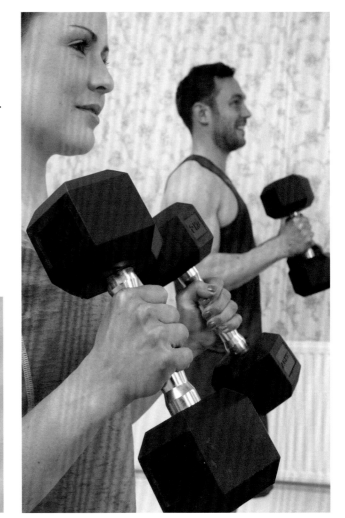

TIPS

Exhale as you curl the weights up, inhale as you lower

For most people, the inward hand position makes this exercise a little easier than standard bicep curls, so you may be able to use a heavier weight

Keep the sides of your elbows pressed into your sides throughout the movement

Perform all stages of the movement in a slow and controlled manner

palm-to-elbow plank

target area
core, arms & chest

equipment
mat

If you mastered the basic plank in Phase I, you're now ready to take it up a gear by adding some movement to the exercise. The good news is this is going to make it less boring to do and the even better news is that it's going to be even more effective in flattening and firming the belly. It does make it harder, of course, but that's all part of the fun!

1 Set up in the same way as a standard plank (p. 101) balancing on your elbows (which should be placed under shoulders) and the balls of your feet, ensuring that your body is straight from head to heels.

2 While keeping your body tight and rigid, place your right palm onto the mat beneath your shoulder and straighten the arm. Then do the same on the left, rising into a straight-arm plank.

3 Now return to the starting position by replacing your right forearm and then your left. This is one repetition. Repeat starting with the left arm.

TIPS

Do not attempt this exercise until you can hold the standard full plank for at least 30 seconds

Exhale as you raise the body into the straight arm plank, inhale as you lower

Maintain straight body alignment and keep the core tight throughout

Palms should be placed on the mat below the shoulders as should the elbows when returning to the low position

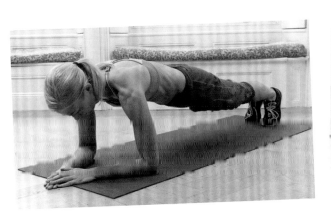

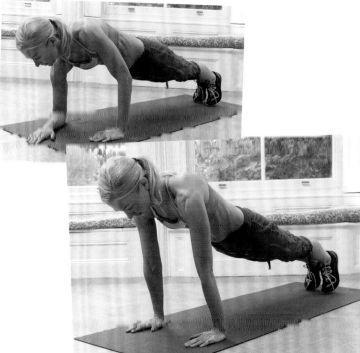

Show the world you can

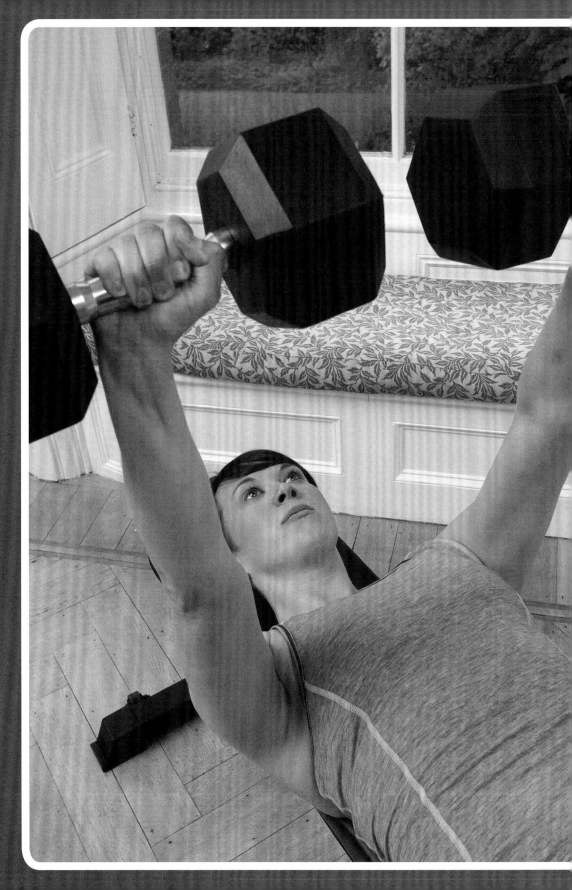

Phase III workout schedule

Congratulations on reaching the final phase of the Fat Burn Revolution!

If you are following the standard schedule you only have four weeks to go and then you'll have finished the entire programme.

By now, your healthier habits have probably become more natural to you as you have repeatedly practised them and regular exercise has become an established aspect of your life. Your tastes in food may have started to change and sugar and carb cravings may have eased or perhaps even disappeared entirely. You can look forward to increases in these benefits and many more rewards during Phase III as the commitment, energy and time you continue to put in pays dividends.

Once again, in Phase III you have three Metabolic Workout sessions. This time they are: arms and shoulders; legs and glutes; chest, back and core.

The Plyo Blaze workout uses some of the plyometric moves you already know from the Total Body Blast and Metabolic Blaster workouts bringing them together in a single fast-paced, calorie massacre of a session! This workout is intense, but short. You get out what you put in with this type of training, so give it your all and you can look forward to fantastic results both in terms of improved fitness and speed and, of course, accelerated fat loss.

You also now have a new supplementary workout, the Belly Shred. This combination of exercises will strengthen and shape your abs and core muscles. Do Belly Shred regularly and you are going to love what happens to your abdominal area! You can perform this workout every other day if you want to, but you will most likely get some soreness after the first couple of times you do it and you should not repeat the workout until this has passed.

Belly Shred takes about 20 minutes to complete and can be done immediately after one of your other workouts or your 30 minutes' steady state activity. It could also be done as a session on its own, but for this you will need to warm up for 10 minutes beforehand.

Here is the standard recommended schedule for Phase III:

day	workout
1	Metabolic Workout 1 – chest, back & core plus Belly Shred
2	Plyo Blaze
3	Metabolic Workout 2 – arms, shoulders & core plus Belly Shred
4	Rest or Phase III Furnace Workout
5	Metabolic Workout 3 – legs, glutes & core plus Belly Shred
6	Phase III Furnace Workout
7	Rest

After performing your warm-up and the upper-body dynamic stretches, start with the warm-up combo. Each of the exercises should be performed once for the stated number of repetitions. You can then move straight onto superset #1. You do not need to start with a warm-up for every set in this workout as the stretches and warm-up combo should be enough preparation.

Perform the upper body static stretches at the end of the session.

warm-up combo

- Alternating bent-over row (p. 159) x 20
- Chest fly (p. 125) x 10
- Good mornings (no weights) (p. 108) x 10

Perform once through doing each of the three exercises using a comfortable weight (around ¾ of your top weight).

1-minute rest

Start superset #1

superset #1

- Bent-over row (p. 90) x 10
- Single arm chest fly (p. 160) x 10

First full set then 1-minute rest

Second full set then 1-minute rest

Move on to next superset

superset #2

- Chest press (p. 126) x 10
- Double back extension (p. 161) x 10

First full set then 1-minute rest

Second full set then 1-minute rest

Move on to next superset

superset #3

- Reverse grip bent-over row (p. 162) x 10
- Straight leg deadlift (p. 163) x 10

First full set then 1-minute rest

Second full set then 1-minute rest

Move on to core sculpt combo

core sculpt combo

- Wood chop (p. 140) x 15 one side
- Saxon side bend (p. 143) x 10 alternating sides
- Wood chop (p. 140) x 15 opposite to first side
- Saxon side bend (p. 143) x 10 alternating sides

Complete once

Got some energy left in the tank? You have the optional extra challenge of doing one set of each of the exercises again.

Phase III: Belly Shred

This workout targets the core and abdominal muscles. If done regularly, with correct form, these exercises will help you achieve a flat, toned abdominal area, as well as strengthening and protecting your back.

The session takes around 20 minutes to complete.

The abdominal muscles tend to adapt and recover quite quickly, so don't worry if you can't do very much at first, you will see good progress over the next four weeks.

You will feel the burn in your abs and possibly in your upper legs too. This is nothing to be concerned about: it is very beneficial to train these muscles to work together in synergy.

(However, if the feeling goes beyond discomfort into pain then you should and seek advice from a medical professional.)

format

If you are not doing this workout straight after one of the other workouts in the programme, perform a 10-minute warm-up before you begin.

Go through all exercises once, taking a 30-second rest between each set of two.

It is likely that you may not be able to do the full number of reps or hold the positions for a full minute at first. That's fine, just do as much or hold as long as you can and aim to increase a little a bit over time working up to the full amount.

If you're new to the static exercises, for example, you might only be able to hold the positions for 30 seconds in the first week of Phase III. Simply make a record of this and try to add 10 seconds on every week to get you to full minute by the final week of the programme.

blast #1
- Gym ball sit-ups (p. 164) x 20
- Lower ab leg lift (p. 111) x 20

30-second rest

blast #2
- V sit-up (p. 165) x 20
- Backwards ball plank (p. 166) x 30 secs to 1 minute

30-second rest

blast #3
- Ball pass (p. 132) x 20
- Side plank (p. 167) x 30 secs to 1 minute

30-second rest

blast #4
- Boat pose (p. 168) x 30 secs to 1 minute
- Stomach vacuum on ball (p. 169) 4 x 5-second holds

Stretch out with at least 5 repetitions of cat (p. 133).

Phase III: Plyo Blaze

 'Get ready to move – this workout is going to rev up your metabolic engine and torch body fat without mercy!'

Plyometric training employs rapid, explosive movements to build strength, power and agility.

This type of exercise annihilates fat and promotes the 'afterburn' effect, which has been accelerating your fat-burning success throughout the Fat Burn Revolution programme.

Improvements tend happen very rapidly with this type of training, and after just a few sessions this workout will give your fitness, energy levels, and metabolism a fierce boost. The whole session can be done in just half an hour, hit it with intense drive and focus and you'll get an incredible fat-burning bang in return for your effort buck!

The exercises are quite advanced, but you are ready to take them on. The workout might be tough at first, but your body will respond to the challenge and it should get a little bit easier every time you do it.

You should push to your maximum, but if you get to a point where your legs get wobbly or you can't keep the correct posture then it is time to rest.

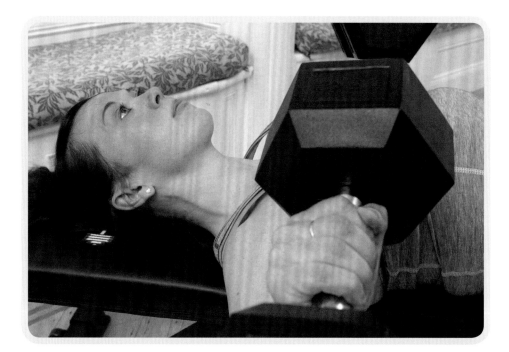

You've come such a long way over the last six weeks and now things are going to get really exciting!

Do not forget to warm up for at least 10 minutes and perform the upper- and lower-body dynamic stretches before doing this workout. Always do both sets of static stretches at the end of the workout too.

format

The workout consists of five sets of two exercises. For the first exercise in each set you should do 15 repetitions, or 30 repetitions for the moves that are performed on alternate sides. The second exercise should be done for 30 seconds. Do the two exercises one after another, without taking a break.

You may not be able to manage the full 30 seconds or 15/30 reps at first. That's fine, just do as much as you can, make a record in your journal of what you did, and try to beat it next time.

After you have done both of the exercises in a set take a one-minute break and then repeat.

When you've done your second set then you can take a one-minute break before moving onto the next set

superset #1
- Broadside bounce (p. 170) x 30 (alternate sides)
- Step-up (fast) (p. 103) x 30 seconds

1-minute rest

Repeat once

superset #2
- Leap-frog jump (p. 171) x 30 (3 hops forward, 3 hops back, x 5)
- Quick step march (p. 172) x 30 seconds

1-minute rest

Repeat once

superset #3
- Squat jacks (p. 173) x 30
- Burpees (p. 102) x 30 seconds

1-minute rest

Repeat once

superset #4
- Squat jump (p. 174) x 15
- Speed bag (p. 175) x 30 seconds each direction

1-minute rest

Repeat once

superset #5
- Split jump (p. 176) x 30 (alternating legs)
- Mountain climbers (p. 177) x 30 seconds

1-minute rest

Repeat once

Phase III: Metabolic Workout 2 | arms, shoulders & core

After performing your warm-up
and dynamic stretches, start with the warm-up combo. Each of the exercises should be performed once for the stated number of repetitions. You can then move straight onto superset #1. You do not need to start with a warm-up for every set in this workout as the stretches and warm-up combo should be enough preparation.

warm-up combo
- Alternating hammer curls (p. 148) x 10 – to perform, switch arms with each repetition
- Alternating shoulder press (p. 93) x 10 – to perform, switch arms with each repetition
- tricep push-up (p. 139) x 10

Perform once through doing each of the three exercises using a comfortable weight (around ¾ of your top weight).

1-minute rest

Start superset #1

> 'Got some energy left in the tank? You have the optional extra challenge of doing one set of each of the exercises again before relaxing with your static stretches.'

superset #1
- Bicep curl (p. 94) x 10
- Tricep kickback (p. 95) x 10

First full set then 1-minute rest

Second full set then 1-minute rest

Move on to next superset

superset #2
- Shoulder press (p. 93) x 10
- Diamond push-up (p. 145) x 10

First full set then 1-minute rest

Second full set then 1-minute rest

Move on to next superset

superset #3
- Concentration curls (p. 178) x 10
- Tricep dips (p. 144) x 10

First full set then 1-minute rest

Second full set then 1-minute rest

Move on to next superset

shoulder shaper combo
- See p. 179

First full set then 1-minute rest

Second full set and cool down

Phase III: Furnace Workout

5-minute warm-up

Begin performing your chosen activity at an easy,
low-intensity pace and gradually build up until
you're at 6–7/10 effort over at least five minutes.

This time you're going to be giving the intervals
100% and putting 10/10 effort into each blast. It's
only for seconds though and that minute rest soon
comes. Dig in eight times and you're done.

effort blasts

- Exercise at maximum intensity for 30 seconds
- Exercise at recovery pace for 60 seconds

Repeat x 8

5-minute cool-down

Continue at an easy pace for five minutes while
your heart rate comes down and breathing slows.

stretch

Stretch any muscles that feel tight or any that you
felt a burning sensation in during the session.

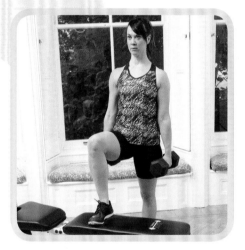

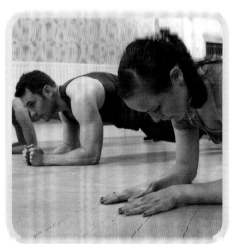

After warming up and performing your lower-body dynamic stretches, start with the warm-up combo. Each of the exercises should be performed once for the stated number of repetitions. You can then move straight onto superset #1. You do not need to start with a warm-up for every set in this workout as the stretches and warm-up combo should be enough preparation.

Finish by performing the lower-body static stretches.

warm-up combo

- Shallow squat x 15 – this exercise is like a normal squat, but you don't come down as low
- Shallow lunge x 15 – this exercise is like a normal lunge, but you don't come down as low
- Calf raise (p. 110) x 15

Perform these exercises without weights before moving onto superset #1

superset #1

- Ball leg curl (or standard squat if you don't have your gym ball handy) (p. 135) x 15
- Wide leg squat (p. 180) x 15

First full set then 1-minute rest

Second full set then 1-minute rest

Move on to next superset

superset #2

- Elevated split squat (p. 181) x 10 per side
- Weighted hip extension (p. 182) x 15

First full set then 1-minute rest

Second full set then 1-minute rest

Move on to next superset

superset #3

- Single leg wall squat (p. 183) x 1 minute (hold on alternate legs for 10–30 seconds and switch)
- Calf raise (p. 110) x 15

First full set then 1-minute rest

Second full set then 1-minute rest

Move on to next superset

butt blaster combo

- Quadruped bent-leg lift to straight leg lift to diagonal straight leg lift straight leg pulse (p. 184)

Perform each move for 15 reps consecutively on the same leg

Switch legs

Repeat

Cool-down and stretch

Exercise time is 'me time'

alternating bent-over row

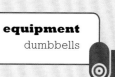
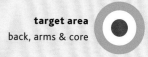
This is a variation of the bent-over row exercise from Phase I. The only difference is that you're going to lift the arms alternately, which is going to require a little bit more coordination, giving the muscles the extra challenge of working independently.

1 Hold a dumbbell in each hand. Plant your feet firmly into the floor, about shoulder-width apart and bend your knees slightly. Then hinge forward from your hips, keeping your back straight and core muscles tight. Let your arms drop down towards the floor holding the dumbbells with palms facing your legs.

2 Lift the left elbow to pull the dumbbell upwards, leaving your right arm dangling down. Your upper arms should be at about a 45-degree angle to your body at the top of the movement.

3 As your left arm comes down, bring the right arm up. That is one repetition.

TIPS

Inhale as you lower the weights and exhale as you perform the pulling movement

Maintain a straight back and keep your neck in-line with your spine, so you'll be looking diagonally down to the floor in front of you

Avoid jerky movements, perform both the pull and release phases in a slow and controlled manner

Do not lift the arm before the other is on the way down

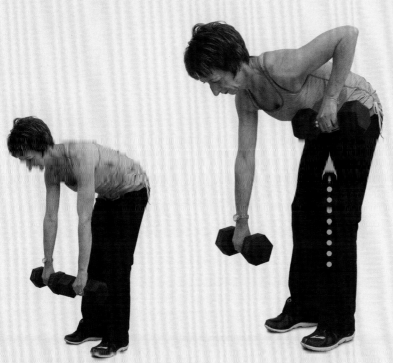

single arm chest fly

This single arm version of the chest fly exercise challenges the chest muscles further, offering even greater lifting and firming benefits for the chest area.

equipment
dumbbells, bench (optional)

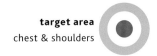

1 Lie face up on your bench or on the floor with knees bent. Hold a dumbbell in one hand. Extend that arm out to your side, keeping a slight bend in the elbow and place the other hand on your hip, elbow pointing out to the side.

2 Keeping the arm extended and elbow slightly bent, bring the dumbbell above the chest, leaving the other arm in place. Hold for a second at the top and then return the arm back out to the side in a slow controlled motion.

3 Perform the exercise for 10 times then repeat with the other arm.

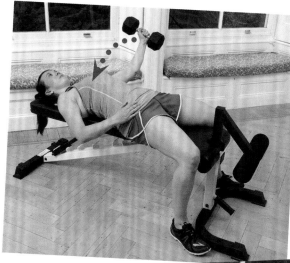

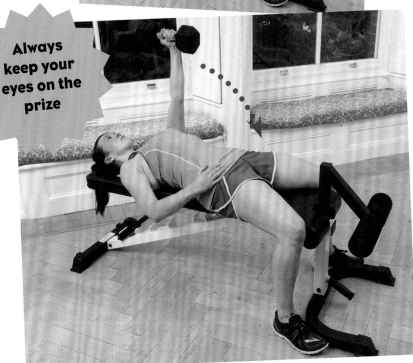

Always keep your eyes on the prize

TIPS

Inhale as you open the arms, exhale as you bring them back in

Do not let the arms drift down below the chest or up beyond the shoulders

Keep your back pressed firmly into the floor/bench and do not allow it to arch up

Really squeeze the pectoral muscles in the chest as you bring the weight up

double back extension

target area
core, lower back & bum

equipment
mat

In Phase I you encountered the leg lift back extension and the arm lift back extension. This move is a mash up of both of those exercises offering double back strengthening and core sculpting benefits.

1 Lie face down on your mat with both of your legs straight and pressed together. Extend your arms straight over your head, palms down.

2 Squeeze the muscles in your lower back as you raise your upper body and your legs off the mat simultaneously, in a slow and controlled movement. Keep your arms and legs straight, knees and ankles stay pressed together. Arms should remain shoulder-width apart, palms facing down.

3 Hold for a second before slowly lowering the chest and legs back down onto the mat. This is one repetition.

TIPS

Breathe in when lifting your body and exhale as you lower

Again, it doesn't matter how high you can lift so long as you feel the muscles working and your technique is correct

Lift to a point that challenges your muscles but is not painful

If you find it too much to lift both legs and arms, try lifting a single arm and leg on opposite sides. Keep alternating sides to complete your reps

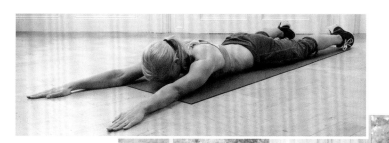

Nothing lifts you
like a good workout.

reverse grip bent-over row

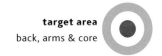

This is another variation of the bent-over row. This time you'll simply be changing the position of your hands to work the bicep muscles in the upper arms a little harder at the same time as shaping the upper back and activating the core muscles.

1 Hold a dumbbell in each hand. Plant your feet firmly into the floor, about shoulder-width apart, bend your knees slightly then hinge forward from your hips, keeping your back straight and core muscles tight. Let your arms drop down towards the floor, holding the dumbbells with palms facing away from your legs.

2 Squeezing your shoulder blades together, pull the dumbbells up towards your lower ribcage. Your upper arms should be at about a 45-degree angle to your body at the top of the movement.

3 Lower the weight back down in a slow and controlled motion to return to the starting position.

TIPS

Inhale as you lower the weights and exhale as you perform the pulling movement

Keep your back straight and neck in-line with your spine, you should be looking diagonally down to the floor in front of you

Maintain control as you move, go slowly and don't jerk the weights up and down

Really concentrate on squeezing the muscles of the upper back to draw the weights in towards you

Soon you will be the one inspiring other people to join the Fat Burn Revolution.

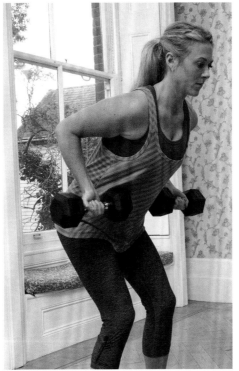

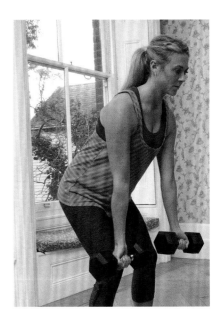

straight leg deadlift

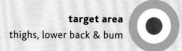

equipment
dumbbells (optional)

Good form is more important than ever when doing this exercise, so start out with no weights until you've fully mastered the move. Once you can perform this move correctly your body is in for a real treat as it is an excellent move for firming and strengthening the back of the body, especially the thighs and buttocks. It works a lot of very large muscles, so it's a great fat burner too.

1 Stand straight and tall, head up, looking forward, feet shoulder-width apart. If you're using weights hold a dumbbell in each hand in front of your thighs, palms facing the body. Otherwise, place your hands on your hips, elbows out.

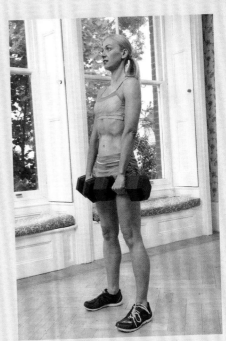

2 Keep the back very straight, core tight, and hinge forward at the hips. You are aiming to get your back parallel to the floor eventually, but depending on your flexibility you may not be able to get that low. Only come down to a point where you feel a comfortable stretch in the back of your thighs. If you're holding dumbbells keep your arms straight and close to your legs as you lower.

3 Squeeze the buttocks as you slowly return to the upright position, always maintaining a very straight back.

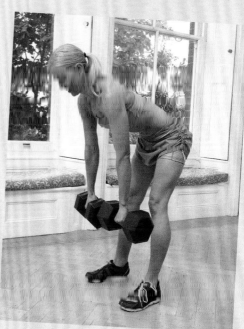

TIPS

Breathe in as you lower your body, breathe out when returning to the starting position

Maintain a straight back, tight core and keep your neck in-line with your spine throughout the exercise

Even if you can get comfortably get down low, do not allow the weights to touch the ground

Perform this exercise in a very slow and controlled manner, never jerk or use momentum

gym ball sit-up

The sit-up is a progression of the basic crunch exercise you encountered in Phase I. You'll be adding further spice to the mix in this version by performing the move on your gym ball. You'll feel this mainly in the front of your tummy, but your bum, thighs and entire midsection will also be getting a workout as you engage muscles across the body to keep you stable.

1 Sit upright on your gym ball with both feet firmly planted on the floor. Now walk your feet away from the ball, slowly lowering your back onto the ball as it rolls beneath you, until your hips and mid-back are resting on the ball. Your knees should be about shoulder-width apart, bent at roughly 90 degrees, and your feet should be parallel. Place your hands behind your head as in the crunch exercise.

2 Lift your upper body to bring yourself into an upright sitting position on the ball. Concentrate on your abdominal muscles contracting as you come up.

3 Lower your body back onto the ball slowly and gently, keeping the feet and knees in place. That is one repetition.

TIPS

Breathe out as you lift and inhale as you lower

Do not pull yourself up with your arms. Your hands are behind your head only to gently support the weight of it and take pressure off your neck

Do not let the elbows drift inward, concentrate on keeping them pointing out to the sides

Aim to keep the movement continuous, however if you start slipping off the ball you may need to stop and correct your position

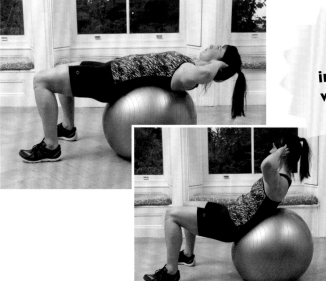

When in doubt, workout!

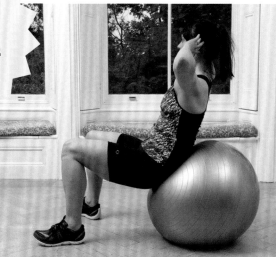

v sit-up

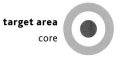

The V sit-up is one of my favourite abdominal exercises because it works the upper and lower parts of the abs hard as well as being a great fat-burning move. You may find this one tough at first, but keep trying and your body will respond by strengthening and sculpting the abdominal area.

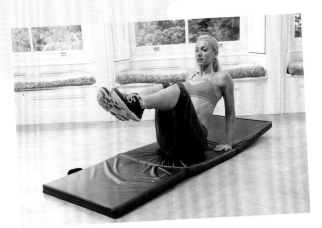

1 Sit upright on your mat with your knees bent, feet down. Take a breath in and, as you exhale, engage your abdominal muscles squeezing them in tight. Now, keeping your back very straight and your abs contracted, lean backwards a little and place your palms down on the mat just behind your hips to help support yourself in this position. Keeping your legs together, lift your feet up from the mat so the lower legs are parallel to the floor. Start by keeping the knees bent and as you get more advanced work towards straightening the legs. Always aim to create a V shape between your thighs and upper body.

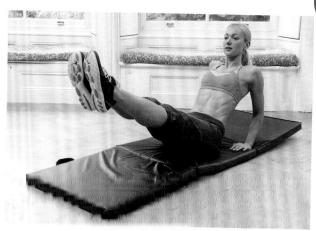

2 Now, keeping your back straight and the lower legs parallel to the floor make the V shape narrower by bringing the body and thighs together. Exhale as you do this.

3 Open the 'V' once again by simultaneously leaning back with the upper body and moving the legs away. Inhale as you do this

TIPS

Don't let your back bend, focus on keeping it straight, core tight

To increase the intensity, perform the exercise with your arms extended straight up over your head and your legs straight

Correct breathing is important, exhale as you bring the thighs and chest together, inhale as you lean back

Keep your neck in line with your spine and be careful not to jut the head forward

backwards ball plank

You practised doing the plank with your elbows on your gym ball in Phase II, now we're going to up the belly-busting ante even more by holding the position with your feet on the ball!

target area
core & lower back

equipment
gym ball, mat

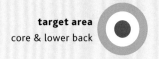

1 Get on the mat on all fours with your gym ball behind you.

2 Place one foot at a time on top of the ball, coming into a straight arm plank position. Your palms should be down on the mat supporting your weight at one end and the tops of your feet should be on the ball at the other end. Once again, ensure your body is in a straight line from head to feet.

3 Hold the position as still as you can for as long as you can before slowly returning one knee at a time to the mat.

TIPS

As always in plank, ensure you don't hold your breath

Hold the core muscles tight and squeeze the bum

The further on the ball your feet are placed the easier this will be

You may find it easier to do this with bare feet

Your body hears everything your mind says, so stay positive.

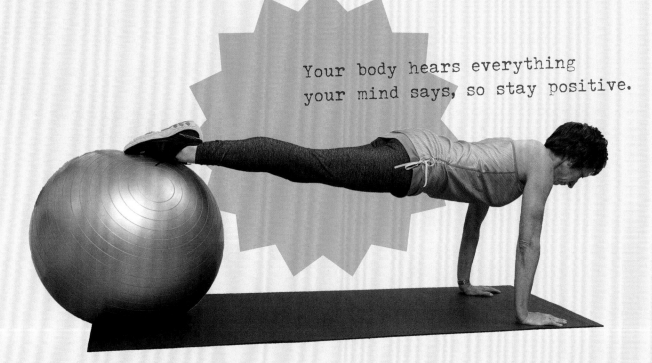

side plank

This is a great move for whittling the waist. You'll also be working the whole abdominal area and your bum while holding this simple yet impressive static pose. Once mastered, this is a good exercise to pull out of the bag when you're out to show off your skills to admiring onlookers!

1 Lie on your left side with your body in a straight line from heels to head. Place your left elbow directly under your shoulder.

2 Bracing your abdominal muscles, lift your hips and legs and come up to support yourself on the elbow, keeping that straight line from heels to head. Now your weight should be resting on the elbow and the side of your left foot.

3 Squeeze your bum and keep your core tight as you hold the position as still as possible before gently returning your body to the mat. Repeat on the opposite side.

target area
core & bum

equipment
mat

TIPS

Keep breathing at the same time as holding your core tight – take shallow breaths from the top of your chest

Maintain straight body alignment and hold the position as still as you can

Once you have mastered this position you can place the palm on the mat and straighten the supporting arm

To advance the exercise further, straighten the supporting arm and raise the top leg

Advanced techniques

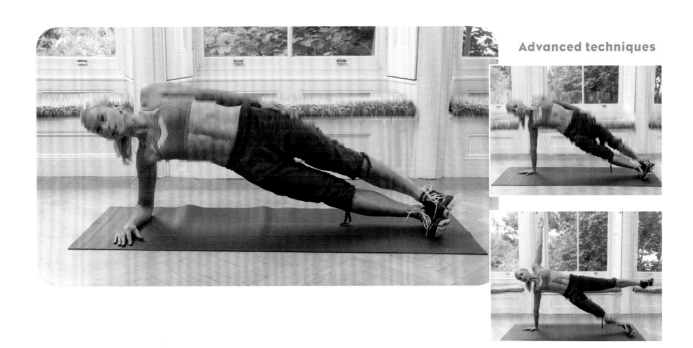

boat pose

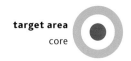

Boat pose is a fantastic static exercise used in yoga to strengthen and tighten the whole of the midsection, especially the abs and lower back. It also improves posture and is great training for core control, which will improve the way you move and perform in all physical activities.

1 Start by sitting up very straight with your knees bent, feet on the floor. Hold onto the sides of your thighs, just under your knees, with your hands. Taking your time as you find your balance, lean back slightly and lift your feet up from the floor so you're balancing on your sit bones.

2 Keeping your back straight and core tight, slowly release your grip on your thighs and lift your arms a little so they're parallel to the floor.

3 Either hold this position or, if you're ready for more of a challenge, straighten the legs as much as you can. You're aiming to eventually get into a posture which forms a V shape, with straight legs at a right angle to your straight body.

TIPS

Do not hold your breath. Keeping your core tight, take shallow breaths from the top of your chest

Hold the position as still as you can

Ideally, your thighs and back should both be at a 45-degree angle to the floor, with a 90-degree angle between them

If it's too challenging at first, keep holding onto your thighs and practise releasing the arms for a few seconds at a time

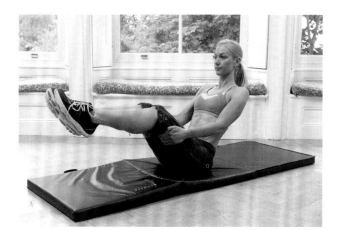

It never gets easier; forget about easy, you just get stronger and fitter.

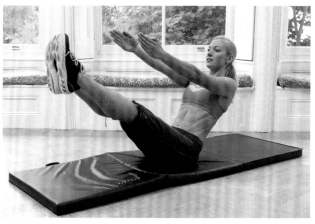

stomach vacuum on ball

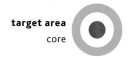

This is a really handy exercise to learn because once you've got the hang of it you can work on your abs virtually anywhere – on the way to work, standing in a queue, even while you're sitting on the sofa watching TV. When doing these as part of a workout, I prefer to perform them on a gym ball to give the core the extra challenge of keeping you stable during the exercise.

1 Sit up straight with your hips on top of your stability ball. Both feet should be firmly planted on the ground, shoulder-width apart. Place your hands on your hips.

2 Relax the belly and take a deep breath in, filling the lungs entirely. Now exhale the breath out, pulling in the abdominals as tightly as you can, squeezing the tummy and waist inwards as you empty every bit of air from your lungs.

3 Hold for a few seconds before inhaling and taking a few breaths to recover. Hold the breath, just for five seconds at first and if that is comfortable try adding on a few more seconds until it is a challenge. Do not hold the breath for too long for obvious reasons!

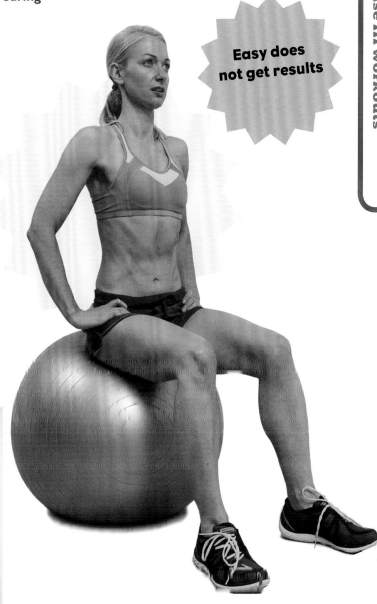

Easy does not get results

TIPS

It you start to feel dizzy or nauseous stop immediately

Sit directly upright with a very straight back, head up, chest proud

Pull in your belly as tightly as you possibly can on the out-breath, think about a tight belt pulling you in or try to squeeze your belly button back into your spine

This exercise can also be performed while standing, kneeling, lying or on all fours

broadside bounce

This is a great fat-burning move that will get you faster on your feet as well as firming up the whole lower body. I've put this exercise at the beginning of the Plyo Blaze workout because it will help get you prepared for the explosive moves that follow.

1 Stand tall with your feet a little wider than your shoulders, arms by your sides.

2 Bending the right knee a little, raise your left knee up across the front of your body. Hold the position, just for a second, engaging the abdominal muscles. Then take a wide sideways hop over onto the left foot. As you land on the left, raise the right knee up.

3 Repeat the movement on alternate sides moving as fast as you can while maintaining good form.

TIPS

Keep the knee of the standing leg slightly bent

The hips, shoulders and head should stay facing forward, back straight

Think about 'crunching' the abdominals as you raise the leg

Get as much height as you can as you leap to the side

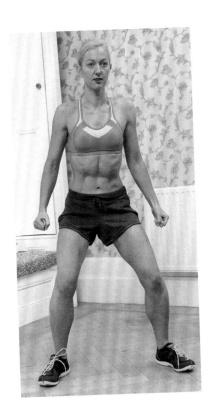
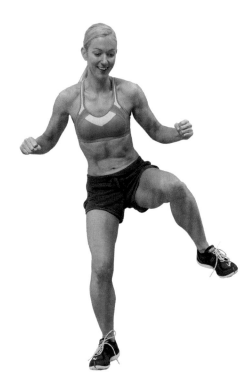
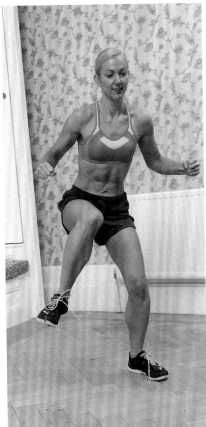

leap-frog jump

This ballistic booty-enhancing move may be brutal, but if you aim to carve yourself a beautiful butt, this exercise is bang on. Get ready to literally work your ass off!

1 Sit back into a squat position with your arms at your sides.

2 From the bottom of the squat, leap forward, bending your elbows and raising your arms to chest level.

3 Come down into the squat position again as you land. Then repeat but this time leap backwards.

TIPS

Remind yourself of the correct way to perform a squat (p. 109) before trying this exercise

Land with the balls of the feet first, knees bent

Jump from the bottom of the squat. Do not stand up and then jump

Keep your back straight and head up at all times

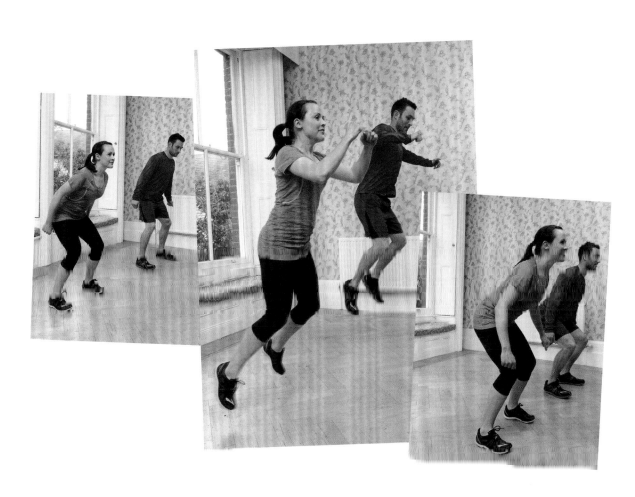

quick step march

Easy to master, tough to perform, the quick step march is a fast-paced move with excellent fat-burning potential.

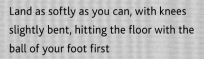

1 Stand tall in front of your step or bench with your hands by your sides, feet hip-width apart. Now step up onto your platform with your right foot. Bend your left knee a little as you prepare to begin.

2 Start the exercise by quickly switching the position of your legs. So you're hopping up and placing the left foot on the platform at the same time as moving the right foot down to the floor.

3 Keep switching the legs for the duration of the exercise without pausing.

TIPS

Your knees, ankles and feet should be pointing forward at all times

You should keep your back straight and core tight, but it is OK to lean forward a little to help you balance as you switch legs

Land as softly as you can, with knees slightly bent, hitting the floor with the ball of your foot first

You can pump your arms at your sides to help keep momentum in this exercise

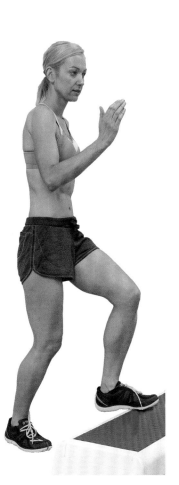

Don't waste time thinking about it, just lace up your shoes and get moving.

squat jack

Get ready to feel the burn in your bum and thighs as you put your booty to work with this metabolism-boosting move.

1 Start standing tall with a straight back, head up, arms by your sides.

2 Jump your feet wide apart, bending the knees as you come down into a wide squat position. At the same time raise your arms out and up as in Jumping Jacks.

3 Jump your feet back together and bring your arms by down to your sides. This is one repetition.

TIPS

Land as softly as you can, balls of the feet first

Keep your back straight, core tight, head up

Land with the feet pointed slightly out as in the wide leg squat exercise and make sure the knees track out over the feet

Only raise your arms to a height that feels comfortable

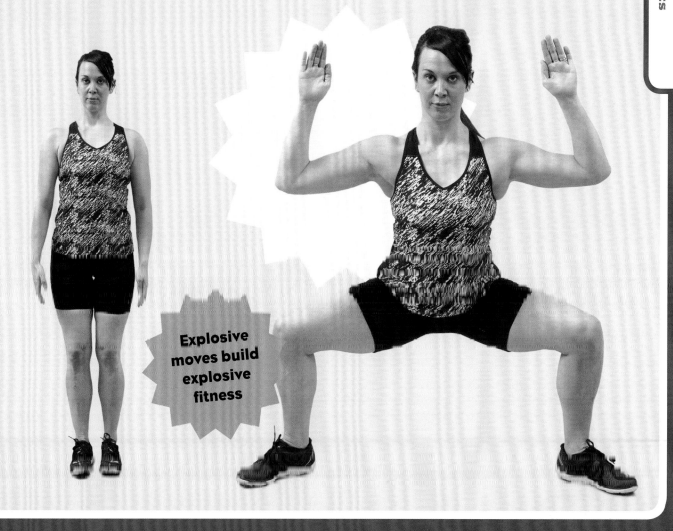

Explosive moves build explosive fitness

squat jump

Squat jumps fire up lots of large muscle groups, but the thighs and bum are the main players in this explosive move. As well as torching a ton of calories, squat jumps build strength and power in the lower body. It's not an easy one, but when you master it and become able to get a lot of air between your feet and the ground, it feels amazing.

1 Get into a squat position (as in the squat exercise, p.109), arms by your sides.

2 From the bottom of the squat push the feet into the floor to jump up off the ground, raise your arms to the ceiling as you leap up.

3 Land as softly as you can, with knees bent, planting the balls of your feet first, then come back down into the original squat position to repeat the movement.

Jump for the moon and you might just land on a star.

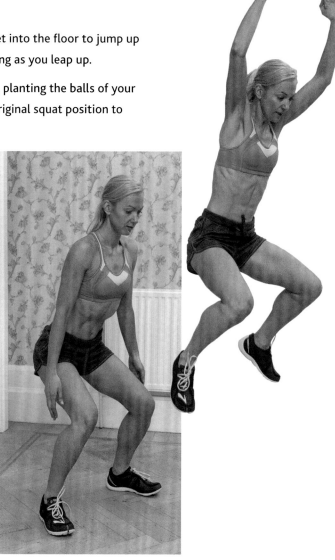

TIPS

You should only attempt this move once you are proficient in the standard squat exercise

Keep your core tight and your back straight

Jump up quickly, initiating the leap from the squat position (do not stand up and then jump)

Move as fast as you can, but do not sacrifice good technique for speed

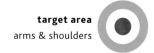

speed bag

This exercise mimics the speed-bag training boxers use to teach their arms to move quickly. We're using it because it's a great fast-paced upper body move to do while our legs get a bit of a rest. You probably don't have a real speed bag to practise with, but that's OK, an imaginary one will do fine.

1 Stand in front of your imaginary speed bag, clench your fist and bring them up to eye level, one just in front of the other. Let your elbows point out to the sides.

2 Pretend to repeatedly punch the speed bag by rotating your fists, as fast as you can, around each other in a small circle. Ensure the arms don't drop down as they get tired, keep the fists up at eye level and don't slow down.

3 Continue the movement for 30 seconds in one direction then rotate the arms in the opposite direction for another 30 seconds.

TIPS

Keep your back straight and your head up

Move your fists as fast as you can

Do not take your eyes off your hands

Make sure your fists don't drift in too close to your head – you do not want to hit yourself in the face!

Show your body how much you want this

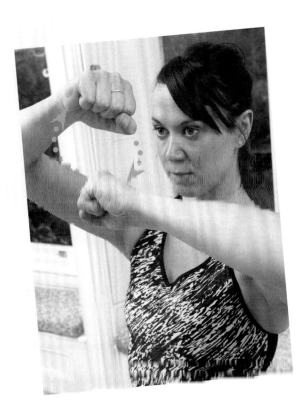

split jump

Split jumps stoke up the metabolism by working the large muscles in the thighs and buttocks hard and fast. You'll be building explosive power as well as firming and strengthening the whole lower body in this move, which is a progression of the split squat.

1 Set yourself up in the split squat position with your arms bent by your sides.

2 From the bottom of the split squat, power up into a jump, switching the position of the legs as you leave the ground.

3 Land as softly as you can with the opposite leg in front. That is one repetition.

TIPS

Exhale as you jump, inhale as you land

Pump your elbows as you jump, landing with the opposite elbow to knee forward

You feet should always point forward as should your knees

Move as quickly as you can while maintaining good technique

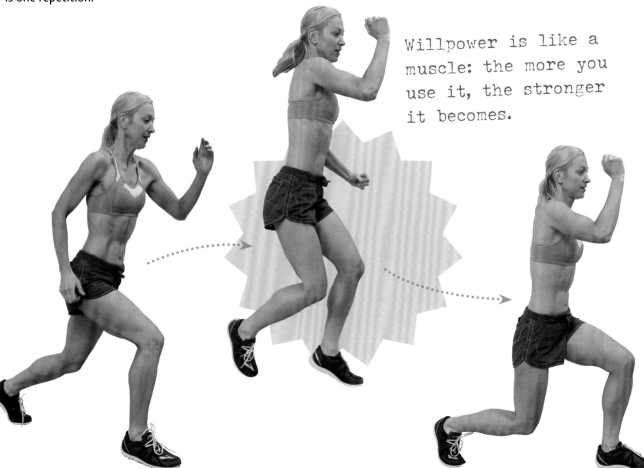

Willpower is like a muscle: the more you use it, the stronger it becomes.

mountain climber

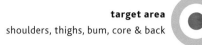

Mountain climbers are fantastic exercise, offering a total body workout in a single 'do anywhere' move. They are hard-core, but if you want to burn body fat these will definitely get you ignited!

1 Start in a straight-arm plank position with your hands on the mat directly under your shoulders, legs extended behind you, balancing on the balls of your feet. Your body should form a straight line from head to heels.

2 Bring your right knee towards your chest and let the foot tap the ground before quickly extending it back and bringing the left foot up to tap the ground.

3 Start off slowly, but once you've mastered the technique pump the legs as fast as you can, bringing the knee up at the same time as the opposite leg thrusts back out behind you so that both feet are off the ground during the transition.

TIPS

Keep your back straight, core tight, neck in-line with spine

If you find this difficult because you don't have enough flexibility in your hips, place your hands on a step or other sturdy platform to elevate the upper body

Aim to stop your hips rising up as you switch legs

The palms should stay flat on the ground throughout the exercise

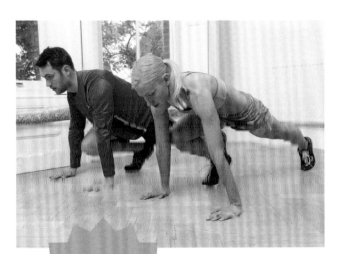

Work it for your 'After' photo

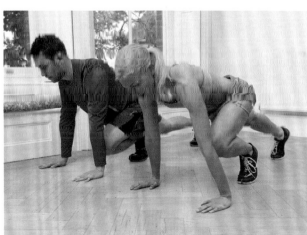

concentration curl

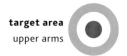
Here's a move to help you win the gorgeous arms race! The concentration curl is a variation of the bicep curl, which isolates the muscle on the front of the upper arm, making it especially effective for firming and defining that area.

equipment
dumbbell

1 Sit on a sturdy bench or chair with your feet and knees wide apart. Holding a dumbbell in one hand, lean forward a little and rest the back of your upper arm on the inside of your leg, just above the knee. Allow the arm to hang down holding the weight with the palm facing inwards. Place the palm of the opposite arm on your other thigh for support.

2 Keeping your back straight and without moving your upper arm, curl the dumbbell upwards to your shoulder. Really squeeze the biceps in the upper arm as you lift and focus on keeping your elbow in place.

3 Lower the dumbbell in a slow and controlled manner back into the starting position. This is one repetition.

TIPS

Breathe in as you lower the weight, exhale as you curl it up

This is a very slow, controlled movement; never swing the weight

The only part of your body that should move is the arm below the elbow; hold everything else still in place

Relax the shoulders and neck

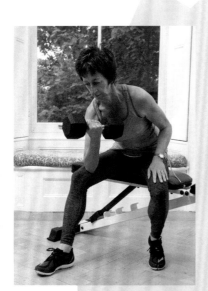

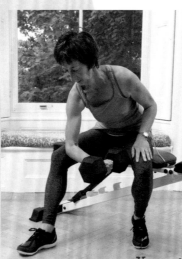

You will only succeed by doing what you need to do, when you feel like it and when you don't.

shoulder shaper combo

Here's a little combination exercise I've cooked up especially to shape, strengthen and sexify your shoulder area. Let's get you sleeveless-top ready!

1 Stand straight and tall with your feet hip-width apart. Start with your arms by your sides holding a dumbbell in each hand with palms facing your body.

2 With just a slight bend at the elbow, slowly raise both of your arms out to the side, bringing the weights up to shoulder level. In a slow controlled motion, lower the weights back down.

3 Rotate your arms to the front of your body so the palms face the front of your thighs. Again, bring the weights up to the level of the shoulders, this time raising the arms straight out in front of you. Slowly lower the arms once more. This is one repetition.

target area
shoulders & upper back

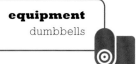

equipment
dumbbells

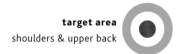

TIPS

Exhale as you lift the weights, inhale as you lower

Make the action slow and controlled, both in the lifting and lowering phases

Keep your arms as straight as you can, with just a slight bend in the elbows

Do not lift the weights above shoulder height

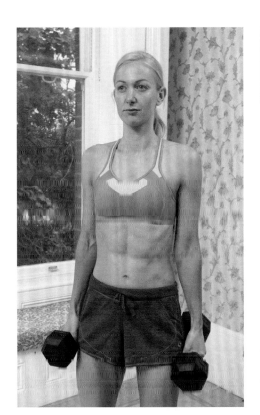

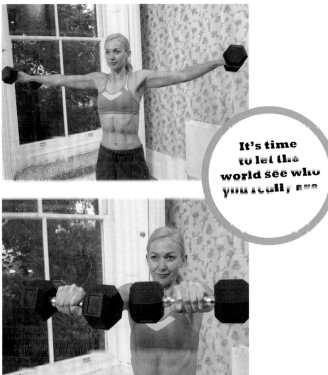

It's time to let the world see who you really are

wide leg squat

This version of the squat exercise works the inner thighs extra hard as well as helping to firm up the whole of the legs and the bum and strengthening the core and lower back.

1 Stand with your feet as wide apart as you can comfortably manage. Try starting out with your feet just beyond shoulder-width apart and if that feels comfortable you can go wider. Feet are slightly turned out. As with standard squats, beginners can start with hands on hips, or to make it a little harder, behind the head, elbows out. Once you've mastered the technique you can hold a dumbbell in each hand.

2 Keeping your back straight and upright, squat down until your thighs are parallel to the floor or as low as you comfortably go.

3 Squeeze your buttocks and push the feet into the floor as you lift your body back to the starting position. This is one repetition.

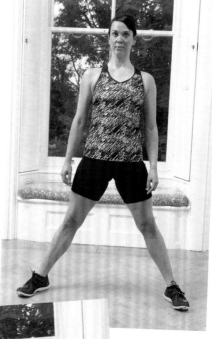

TIPS

You should never feel pain in this exercise: if it hurts your knees, then do not come down as low

---

Inhale as you squat down and breathe out as you raise yourself back up

---

The feet should stay flat on the floor and remain in place througho ut the movement

---

The knees should move in the direction of the feet, do not let them flare in or out

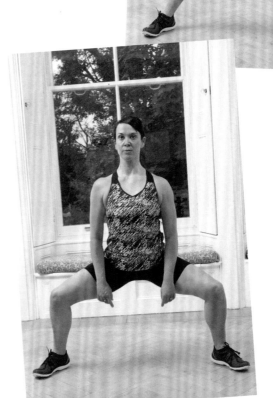

elevated split squat

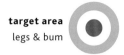

equipment
bench, dumbbells (optional)

This is definitely one of my favourite leg exercises. It's not for beginners – if you have yet to master the standard split squat then stick with that for now. But, if you are ready for this move, you're going to get an excellent workout for all the major muscles of the lower body. This is a great fat-burning move too. Working the legs individually will help you to correct any strength imbalances between right and left, which will generally improve the way you move, reduce the risk of injuries and enhance your lower-body performance.

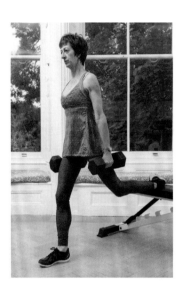

1 You need to set yourself up in the same way as for a standard split squat, but for this exercise you will be placing the back foot on a step, bench or other sturdy surface raised from the floor behind you. Lie the top of your back foot flat down on the surface. You may need to shuffle your front foot forwards a little to get your stance wide enough once the back foot is in place.

2 Concentrate on the front leg and the buttock of that side doing all the work as you lower the hips, the back leg is only there to support you. As with a standard split squat, you are aiming to get the front thigh parallel to the ground, but just go down as low as you can.

3 Slowly push back up pressing the front foot into the floor and letting all the effort come from the front leg. Repeat to complete your reps on that side before switching legs.

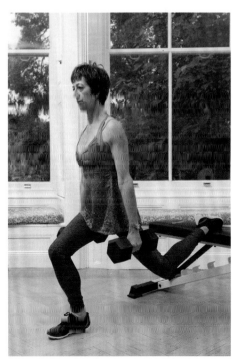

TIPS

Once you're ready to add weights, perform the exercise holding a dumbbell in each hand

Keep your back straight and upright, resist leaning forward as you lower

You front foot should stay facing forward and remain firmly planted on the floor

Do not let your front knee flare out to either side

weighted hip extension

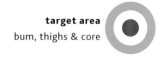

In this version of the hip extension exercise you'll be adding weights to ensure very hot and not-at-all cross buns!

1 As with the standard hip extension, start by lying face-up on your mat with your knees bent, feet flat on the floor. This time you will be upping the ante by holding a pair of dumbbells or a weight plate over your hips.

2 Keeping your feet flat and your shoulders resting on the mat, gently lift your hips as high you can, squeezing your buttocks and keeping your core tight.

3 Hold the position for a second and then slowly lower the hips back down onto the mat. This is one repetition.

TIPS

Exhale as you lift the hips, inhale as you lower

Lift straight up, do not sway or tilt the hips and keeps the knees and feet fixed in place

Lift high enough so that you feel tension in the muscles, but stay lower if it's painful to lift high

If this is easy for you, options to increase the intensity further include lifting a leg or placing the feet on a gym ball as in the Hip Raise on Ball exercise from Phase II

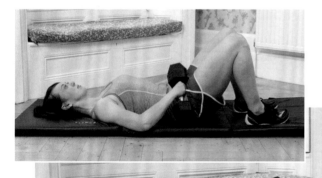

Be proud of how far you've come and all the things you can do now that you couldn't do just a couple of months ago.

single leg wall squat

Remember the delightful wall squat exercise from Phase II? As a special thigh-trimming treat you're now going to perform the exercise on just one leg! You'll thank me later...

1 You need to set yourself up in the same way as for a standard wall squat, but this time your legs, feet and knees should be pressed together.

2 Once in position simply extend one leg forward, keeping the knees together aiming to get the raised leg parallel to the floor. Hold the posture as still as you can. Concentrate on pushing the back into the wall and maintaining the height of the raised leg.

3 Once your time is up, replace the leg and repeat on the other side.

TIPS

Think about breathing from the top of the chest to allow the abs to fully engage

Keep the knee of the non-raised leg over the ankle and the foot pointing forward

Knees and thighs stay pressed together as you raise the leg

Allow the shoulders, neck and arms to relax

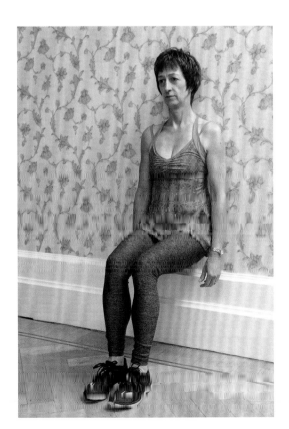

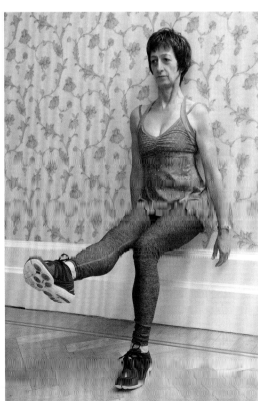

butt blaster combo

Here's a combination of moves to firm, sculpt and tighten your bum and thighs. You should really feel the burn in your bum as you do these. For maximum effect move very slowly and deliberately, really squeezing the muscles as hard as you can.

target area
bum, thighs, lower back & core

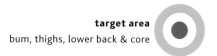

equipment
mat, dumbbell (optional)

1 Start on your hands and knees as in the Superman and airplane exercises. Now, keeping the knee bent at 90 degrees, slowly lift the right leg behind you so the foot rises towards the ceiling. Bring the knee back in, but do not replace it, hover a couple of centimetres above the mat, before raising it again to complete 15 repetitions of that movement.

2 Return the right knee to the mat just for a second before straightening the leg out behind you. Now bring the leg diagonally down to tap the floor with your toe behind the left foot, before lifting it up again in the horizontal position in-line with your hip. Keep the leg straight as you repeat this movement 15 times.

3 Keep the leg extended straight behind you at hip level and lift it just a little higher (about 5cm) in a pulsing motion directly upwards. Repeat for 15 pulses. Return the knee to the floor before repeating the whole combination with the opposite leg.

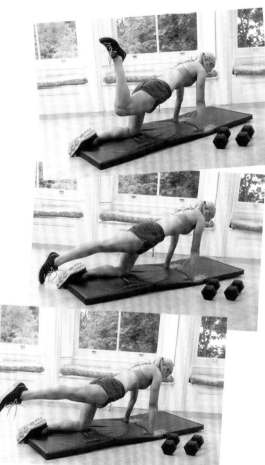

TIPS

Keep your back straight, core tight and neck in-line with spine throughout the exercise

With the exception of the final 'pulse' movement, perform the rest of the exercises in slow motion

You can increase the intensity of the first move, the bent leg lift, by wedging a dumbbell behind your bent knee

Concentrate on squeezing the buttocks and contracting the thighs as tightly as you can

Advanced Step 1 method

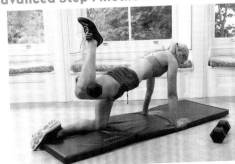

13 vive la revolution

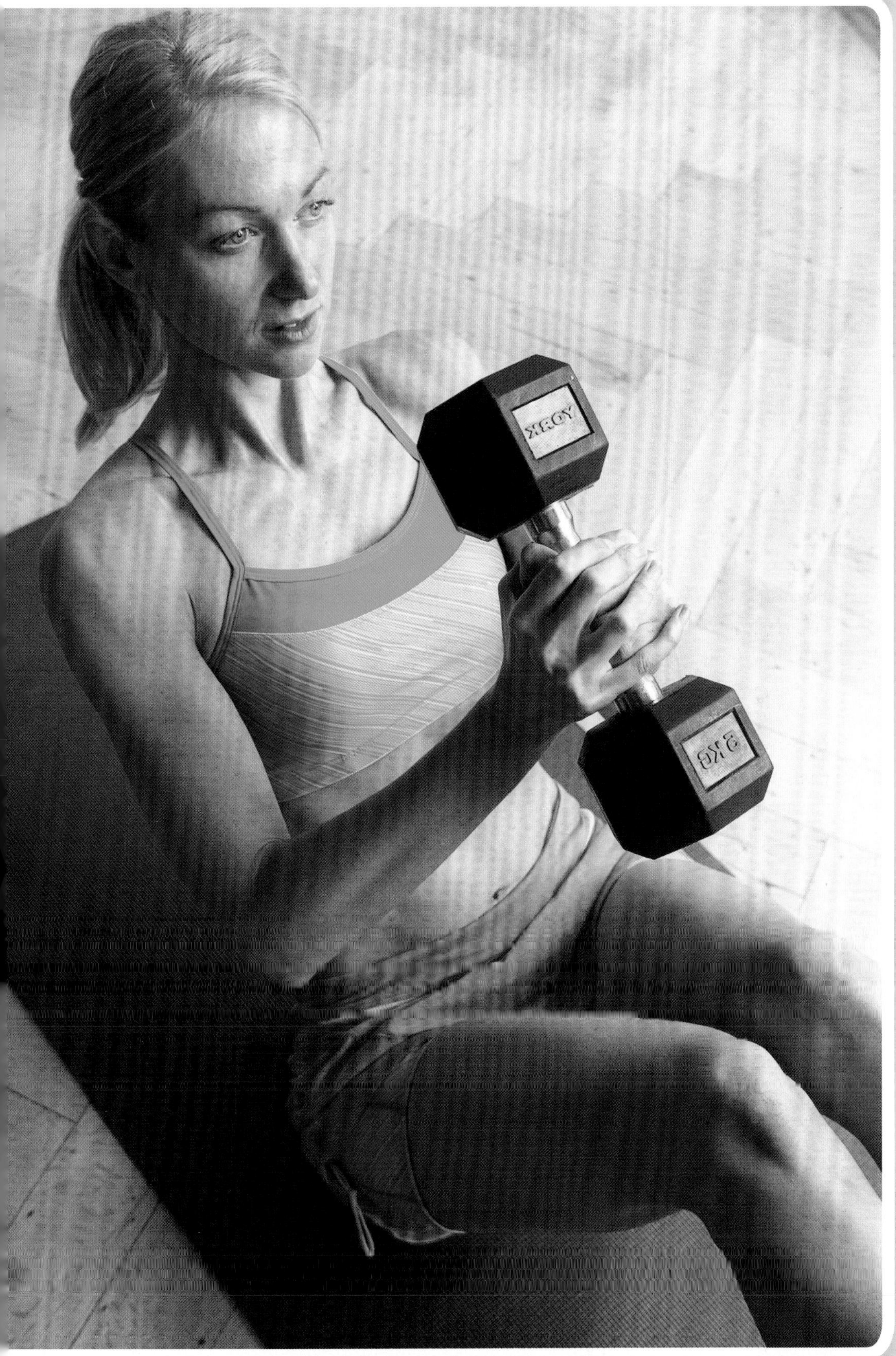

*I*f you're reading this after completing the entire Fat Burn Revolution programme then I just want to say that you have achieved something truly remarkable. Even if you've never felt proud of yourself in your life before, I want you to feel that way now. You've earned it.

You should now be in excellent condition, with your fitness levels well above average. But I'm sure you're feeling benefits that stretch well beyond the physical. You have proven to yourself, and to the world, that you can push beyond your limits and that you have the tenacity and drive to follow on through on your commitments and achieve your goals. You have taken control of your body and your life. Whether you realise it or not, you have now become stronger and more powerful in every way.

The last thing you want now you've discovered how great it feels to be in good shape is to slide backwards and regain fat. I'm sure you have no intention of letting that happen, but I highly recommend you plan a strategy to make sure old habits don't start to creep back in. The best starting point is to come up with a new goal to work towards.

If you're still keen to shed more fat, you now have a clear idea of the rate at which you'll be able to reach your ultimate goal size or body-fat amount. Or if you've got rid of all the fat you want to lose, maybe you'd like to get stronger, in which case you might like to set targets in terms of the weights you like to be able use. Or maybe you'd like to work more on your speed, agility, or explosive fitness? Or perhaps it's a combination. If you've been keeping your journal, you know what level you're at across all those areas, so you're in a great position to set some achievable, but challenging, targets to keep you motived as you move your fitness to the next level.

Now you've built up solid functional, athletic, real-world fitness there's a whole world of exciting fitness challenges and events you could sign up and start training for.

But first of all it might be wise to take some rest and recovery time. The standard 12-week Fat Burn Revolution schedule is intense and requires a lot of commitment to complete. If you've been following that, then your body will benefit from a week off from hard training. I'm not saying you should be totally sedentary for seven days, just bring the intensity right down and have a week where you focus on easy-paced low-impact exercise.

By all means continue with the programme workouts if you want to. Unlike with most programmes you won't experience plateaus if you change the way you train every four weeks – so long as you keep working with challenging weights and pushing yourself to the limit in your sessions, your progress will be

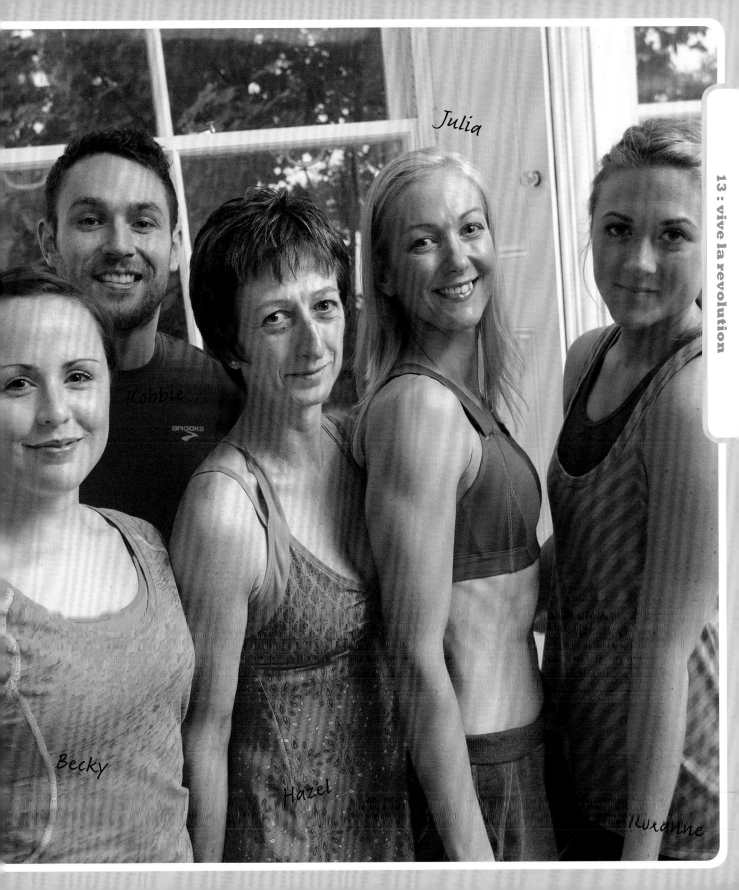

Becky

Robbie

Hazel

Julia

Marianne

on-going. As my pilot testers have discovered, the results of a second round of the programme can be equally impressive. Or you can easily integrate this programme with other types of training, should you wish to try something new. You've learned some of the best exercises it's possible to do over the course of this programme, so you have an excellent repertoire to draw on as you go forward and decide what the best next step should be for your training goals.

The person you were when you turned the first page of this book is gone. Chances are, a lot of their clothes don't fit any more! So, bin them. Now. I highly recommend this as a way to affirm to yourself that you're never going back to being that person again. Plus, buying new well-fitting gear is the perfect reward for all the effort and sweat you've put into sculpting your new shape.

I told you from the very start that the Fat Burn Revolution was not easy, but you took on the challenge and for that you have my utmost respect and admiration. You made a decision that you were no longer going to settle for being out of condition and unhappy with your body. You made a commitment to become fitter, stronger, healthier and leaner. You sweated, you stood firm in the face of temptations and, although I'm sure at times you wobbled and wavered, you did not give up.

At this point I'd like you to spend some time looking back on the journey you've travelled as you've followed the Fat Burn Revolution. Take a look at yourself (literally and metaphorically) and notice the many ways in which you have changed. Remember the times when staying committed to your goals and taking action was hard, but you dug in and got it done anyway? I want you to really take in and appreciate what that says about the person you have now become.

You are amazing. I hope you know that. You have accomplished something outstanding and you are now ready to go forward and experience even greater triumphs. One result of which will doubtless be that you will become an inspiration to others.

Perhaps you've already noticed how contagious fat loss and fitness can be?

I dedicate most of my time to sharing what you've learned during this programme with as many people as I can and I hope you'll now join me in the crusade to share the secrets to a Fat Burn Revolution.

Julia

PS You can start doing your bit for the revolution right now by sharing your experiences with the world via my website: juliabuckley.co.uk

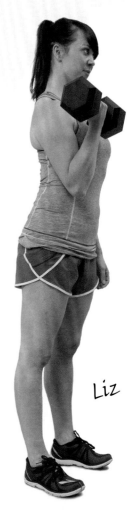

Liz

your **workout** journal

You should record your experiences, daily diet and workout session details in the journals to keep track of your progress. The best thing about keeping a Fat Burn Revolution journal is that it's highly motivational and becomes a record of achievement you can be proud of. For printable versions of the Fat Burn Revolution journal, visit *www.bloomsbury.com/9781408191569*, or visit *juliabuckley.co.uk* for a digital version.

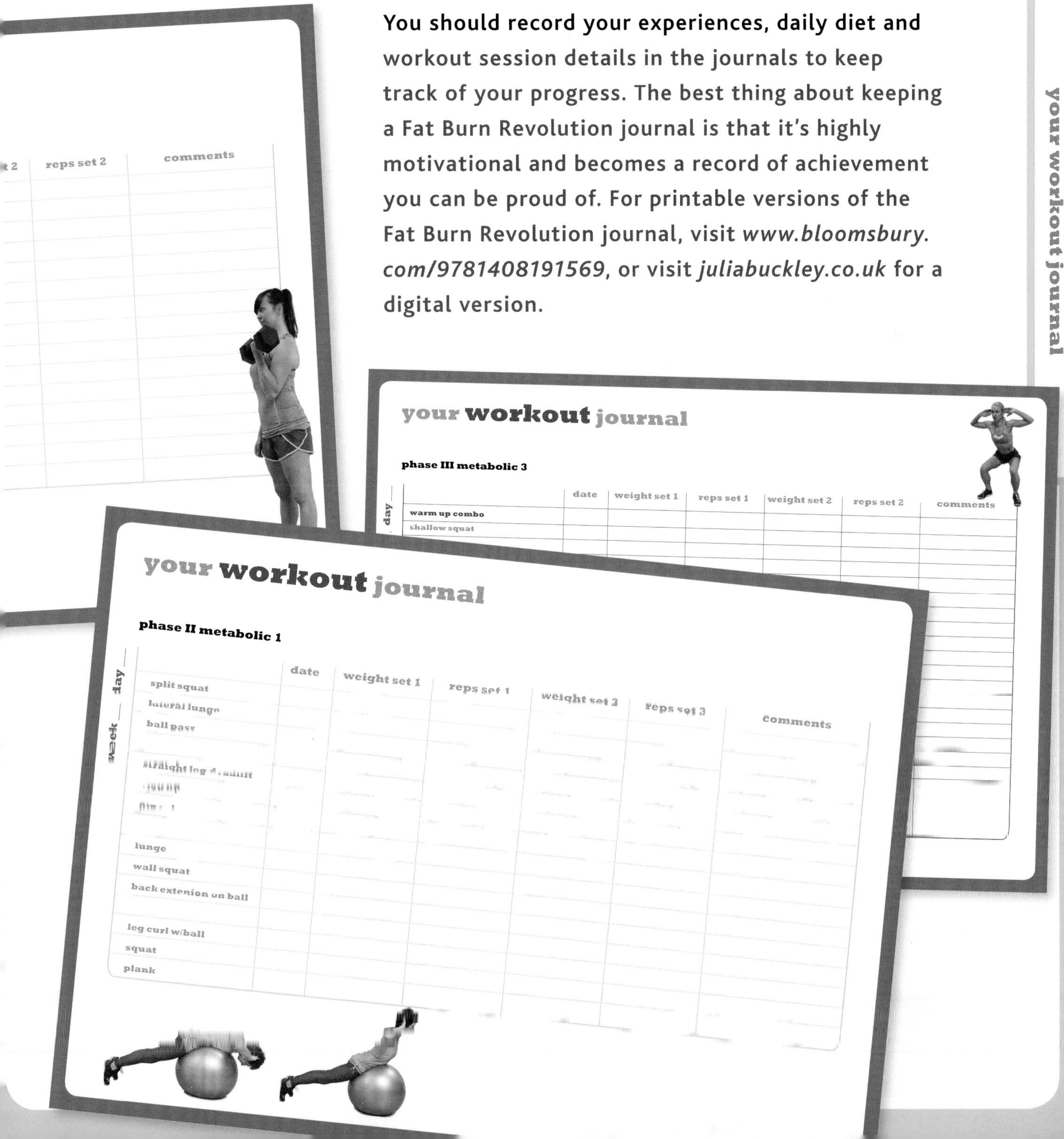

	reps set 2	comments

your **workout** journal

phase III metabolic 3

day		date	weight set 1	reps set 1	weight set 2	reps set 2	comments
	warm up combo						
	shallow squat						

your **workout** journal

phase II metabolic 1

week	day		date	weight set 1	reps set 1	weight set 2	reps set 2	comments
		split squat						
		lateral lunge						
		ball pass						
		straight leg deadlift						
		step up						
		dips						
		lunge						
		wall squat						
		back extension on ball						
		leg curl w/ball						
		squat						
		plank						

index

Entries in **bold** refer to individual exercises and stretches.

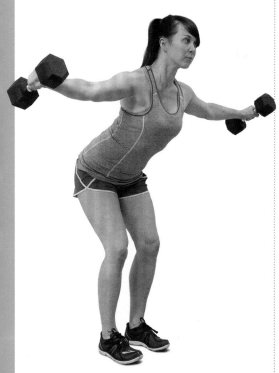

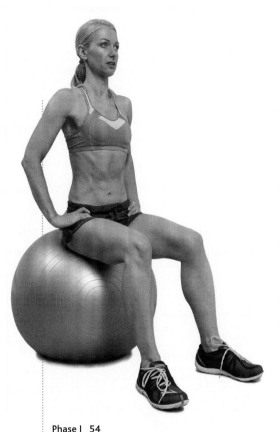